T0046455

TEACHING
YOGA
BEYOND
THE
POSES

TEACHING YOGA BEYOND THE POSES

A PRACTICAL WORKBOOK
FOR INTEGRATING THEMES,
IDEAS, AND INSPIRATION
INTO YOUR CLASS

SAGE ROUNTREE AND ALEXANDRA DESIATO
FOREWORD BY CYNDI LEE,
AUTHOR OF *YOGA BODY BUDDHA MIND*

North Atlantic Books
Berkeley, California

Copyright © 2019 by Sage Rountree and Alexandra DeSiato. All rights reserved. No portion of this book, except for brief review, may be reproduced, stored in a retrieval system, or transmitted in any form or by any means—electronic, mechanical, photocopying, recording, or otherwise—without the written permission of the publisher. For information contact North Atlantic Books.

Published by
North Atlantic Books
Berkeley, California

Cover photo © aninata/Shutterstock.com
Cover design by Rob Johnson
Book design by Happenstance Type-O-Rama
Illustrations by Lasha Mutual, lashamutual.com

Printed in the United States of America

Teaching Yoga Beyond the Poses: A Practical Workbook for Integrating Themes, Ideas, and Inspiration into Your Class is sponsored and published by North Atlantic Books, an educational nonprofit based in Berkeley, California, that collaborates with partners to develop cross-cultural perspectives, nurture holistic views of art, science, the humanities, and healing, and seed personal and global transformation by publishing work on the relationship of body, spirit, and nature.

MEDICAL DISCLAIMER: The following information is intended for general information purposes only. Individuals should always see their health care provider before administering any suggestions made in this book. Any application of the material set forth in the following pages is at the reader's discretion and is their sole responsibility.

North Atlantic Books' publications are distributed to the US trade and internationally by Penguin Random House Publishers Services. For further information, visit our website at www.northatlanticbooks.com.

Library of Congress Cataloging-in-Publication Data

Names: Rountree, Sage Hamilton, author. | Desiato, Alexandra, 1979- author.
Title: Teaching yoga beyond the poses : a practical workbook for integrating
    themes, ideas, and inspiration into your class / Sage Rountree and
    Alexandra DeSiato.
Description: Berkeley, California : North Atlantic Books, [2019]
Identifiers: LCCN 2018048512 | ISBN 9781623173227 (paperback)
Subjects: LCSH: Hatha yoga--Study and teaching. | BISAC: HEALTH & FITNESS /
    Yoga. | BODY, MIND & SPIRIT / Meditation. | SELF-HELP / Motivational &
    Inspirational.
Classification: LCC RA781.7 .R72 2019 | DDC 613.7/046076--dc23
LC record available at https://lccn.loc.gov/2018048512

6 7 8 9 10 11 KPC 25 24 23 22 21

This book includes recycled material and material from well-managed forests. North Atlantic Books is committed to the protection of our environment. We print on recycled paper whenever possible and partner with printers who strive to use environmentally responsible practices.

CONTENTS

Part 3. Creating Themes That Connect

FOREWORD

BY CYNDI LEE

Years ago, when I was teaching a workshop called Yoga Body Buddha Mind in North Carolina, I met Sage Rountree. She was in the front row, which told me that even though her yoga asana practice was full of strength, clarity, and confidence, she wanted to learn more about the invisible parts of this vast thing called yoga. She wasn't just an athletic practitioner, she was a real yogini. After class, she introduced herself to me and gave me a copy of her book, *The Athlete's Guide to Yoga*. From the start, she has had something valuable to say to yogis of all kinds.

Rountree's career as a yoga teacher and author mirrors the path of many hatha yoga teachers: before we go inside, we start with the outside—what we can see and feel. We start with the body. *Hatha* can be translated as "sun and moon," and *yoga* can be translated as relationship or integration. Hatha yoga shows us that when we integrate two oppositional energies in equal measure we come into a sense of wholeness. Hatha yoga offers us this path through the body, but as we practice with our bodies, we also pay attention to what comes up in our mind and hearts. When our yoga experience becomes so profound that it begins to infuse our life with fresh meaning, we often get inspired to share this goodness with others. We become yoga teachers.

Unfortunately, many graduates of teacher-training programs find themselves taking their place in front of the first yoga class they teach and realizing, in a panic, "I don't know what to say about yoga!" Telling people where to put their arms and legs and how to organize the body is just the first half of teaching. As with our own yoga practice, in teaching we also start with the body. We learn to use clear instructional language such as reach, flow, engage, let go, flex, point, lengthen, press down, and lift up.

To evolve from being a yoga instructor to becoming a yoga teacher, one must also include the part about how we notice our thoughts and emotions as we move our bodies. Yoga is not just about doing, it's about experiencing. Teachers want to find ways to verbally articulate these insights that have arisen in their practice. Even more … they want to be able to offer practice experiences to their students in which the words and the movements—the two apparent opposites that together create the whole meaningful experience—are integrated.

Rountree knows this from the arc of her own teaching experience as well as leading numerous teacher trainings. How fortunate for us that she has teamed up with another smart and seasoned yoga teacher, Alexandra DeSiato. These two women have been in the seat of the teacher long enough to know how difficult this second stage of teaching can be. They know that it is natural to feel shy and underconfident, and they also know how to shepherd you through this process. Whether working with athletes who have no time for woo-woo or sharing insights with women going through the very real experience of pregnancy, they have had real opportunities to learn how to speak their truth simply. Then, they trust the practice of yoga to do the rest.

I bet when you take a class from Rountree or DeSiato, they make this look easy. But after forty years of teaching yoga, I can tell you that although it gets easier, it's never easy! Rountree and DeSiato are not just good teachers because they are special (which they are) or because they have years of experience (which they do) but because they have deeply engaged in the yogic practice of *svadyaya*, self-study. In the context of yoga, self-study has a dual meaning. One is taking it upon yourself to deepen your yoga education through reading texts, taking classes, and attending lectures, and the other is learning how to study yourself. This might sound egocentric, but it's really the opposite.

The yogic tradition of self-study invites us to observe our thoughts, feelings, and emotions as a path to freedom from our usual self-centeredness. It's such a relief to understand that whatever thoughts arise will also pass, and this realization helps us recognize that our true center is one of goodness. *Svadyaya* helps us clean out our own closet, so to speak, so we can be more available to our friends and families, and of course, to our students.

Teaching Yoga Beyond the Poses invites you to take a deep dive into *svadyaya*— to bravely look at what comes up in your own yoga practice and then contemplate it and write about it. Rountree and DeSiato guide you in exploring the universality of your personal insights by searching out other's poetic, musical, and spoken expressions of this same common experience. They remind you to honor your lineage by recalling the teachers who came before you and recognizing how the wisdom they shared now lives in you.

One of the many things I really like about *Teaching Yoga Beyond the Poses* is that reading this book is like taking a yoga class. Just as a yoga class deconstructs, explores, and then reconstructs the poses into a whole sequence that is then better understood, this book leads the yoga teacher step-by-step through confusion and obstacles to reach clarity and inspiration. The reader/yoga teacher is given numerous paths toward finding their personal language and a variety of methods for integrating that with instructional language, to finally be able to teach a multi-layered, fully dimensional yoga class.

Rountree and DeSiato start where all teachers start: *what do I do if I am nervous?* I'll tell you a secret: I am nervous before every yoga class I teach. I'm nervous because I care, and I want to do a good job. I care about yoga and even more, I care about all the people who showed up for my class today. It is very clear to me that there is only one reason to be a yoga teacher and that is to be helpful. It's ok to be nervous, but if you find your nervousness is limiting you, Rountree and DeSiato offer you specific methods for practicing speaking, finding role models, playing with language, and learning how to trust that when you do your honest best, that's enough.

The second thing I really like about *Teaching Yoga Beyond the Poses* are the many suggested themes that Rountree and DeSiato offer you. Most of the themes are drawn directly from yoga philosophy. This is a powerful reminder that when we get stuck or bored in our practice, when we feel uninspired or unmotivated in our teaching, we can always come home to yoga. We don't have to look outside our own wisdom tradition. This is the message of yoga itself—we don't have to look outside ourselves for validation or knowledge. We can trust our own experiences and understandings. This is also something you can practice.

The thing is that "doing" your own yoga practice is not the same as "doing" your teaching practice. The processes are different, but they both require repetition. Practice triangle pose over and over, and eventually you will be so familiar with it that it becomes part of you. If you want to teach beyond the poses, Rountree and DeSiato tell you to practice saying your words again and again.

What Rountree and DeSiato don't do is tell you what to say. In the tradition of all the very best teachers, when they point to the moon, they make sure you see the moon and not their finger. Throughout this entire workbook, they are modeling what it means to be a yoga teacher. The substantial middle section of the book is a thorough guide for how to find source material for themes and how to make them your own. But just in case you still don't think you are good enough, they also have a chapter called "There Are No Bad Themes."

In the end, this book is more than a yoga class—it's a complete book about the yoga tradition, and I recommend it for anybody who is interested in learning more about yoga. Yoga has been around for centuries, passed down from teacher to student. This kind of oral tradition is called "mouth-to-ear," which means the teacher whispers the secrets into the student's ear. In *Teaching Yoga Beyond the Poses*, Rountree and DeSiato are whispering to you: "Try this. Or this. Take your time. Find out what stories and insights live within you. We'll help you."

Teaching Yoga Beyond the Poses gives you a map to discovering your genuine expression so that you can transmit to your students the message that the best thing they can do is become more themselves. Yoga is never about trying to be a better or different person. Yoga is a map—one that helps you get familiar with yourself in a way that is kind and generous and loving. When you can teach from that place, you will be more than teaching yoga, you will be transmitting to your students the message that they are good as they are.

CYNDI LEE, author of Yoga Body Buddha Mind

PREFACE

Collectively, we have over forty years' classroom experience, both in college English and writing courses and in movement classes, including Spinning, Pilates, and yoga. Those forty years have shown us that the best classes have a clear direction and repeat it often to stay on track, while at the same time allowing for student investigation along the way. While many yoga teachers learn to do this through trial and error, *Teaching Yoga Beyond the Poses* is here to shortcut that process for you, so that you can help your students, and thus your career, more quickly and confidently.

Many of Sage's previous books have focused on how to do poses safely *(The Athlete's Guide to Yoga, The Runner's Guide to Yoga)*, and how to put them together into sequences *(The Athlete's Pocket Guide to Yoga, Everyday Yoga)*. Likewise, our jointly authored *Lifelong Yoga* covers the what and how of choosing poses to support healthy aging and finding ways to modify your practice to suit any stage in life. These books speak directly to students, and teachers have also found them helpful. The book you're holding, instead, speaks directly to teachers, though experienced practitioners who don't teach will also find it helpful. We hope it will inspire you and in turn inspire your students to a deeper connection through yoga.

Maybe you've picked up this book because you want to feel embodied and genuine when you speak to your class. Or perhaps you've picked up this book because while you feel pretty confident about sequencing a balanced and interesting practice, when you try to offer your students tidbits connected to spiritual intention, you freeze up, or your voice shakes, or you hear an echo voice in your head saying things like, "Uh, did you *really* just say that?" Maybe you feel like you aren't wise, present, or ready to lead others to wisdom, presence, or readiness. Maybe you're just tired of saying the same things in a yoga practice and you're ready for a fresh approach. Whatever the reason you're here, we're glad. The starting point is figuring out what your most comfortable, professional, and authentic voice is and speaking from that place. That's our focus in part 1. Along the way, we hope you will follow our journaling prompts. If you are reading this book on paper, don't be afraid to press down and flatten the pages—the book is bound to lie flat with a little pressure. If you're reading in ebook format, write in your favorite journal or create a file to hold your journal responses and theme notes.

In part 2, we offer you fifty-four themes to guide your yoga classes. These are like recipes in a cookbook—you might like to follow them closely at first, then tweak them according to your tastes and the ingredients on hand thereafter. Perhaps you'll wind up cobbling new themes together by combining the templates in unique ways. It's all up to you and what feels most true to your voice and your students' needs.

Once you've grown comfortable exploring our recipes, you can use the templates in part 3 and at http://teachingyogabeyondtheposes.com to create your own themes and notes. We hope you will find years of inspiration in the process.

ACKNOWLEDGMENTS

We wrote this book for you—someone who has been touched by the gifts of yoga and who wants to share them with others. We'd like to acknowledge your generous spirit and wish you all the best on your journey. Thank you for taking the time and effort to make the world a kinder, more connected place.

Thanks also to everyone involved in the creation of this book: our literary agent Linda Konner, our editors Alison Knowles and Ebonie Ledbetter, our copy editor Christopher Church, and the production team at North Atlantic Books. Thanks especially to Lasha Mutual (http://lashamutual.com) for the custom illustrations.

Thanks go to our yoga teacher colleagues—many inspired themes came from our colleagues' classes, yoga philosophy discussions, and through the sharing of playlists and poetry. Thanks go to our students, who encourage our pursuit of meaningful ideas by asking more about the themes we offer in class. Thanks go to our families, in particular, for supporting us in myriad ways and for gifting us with the most important life theme of all: enduring love.

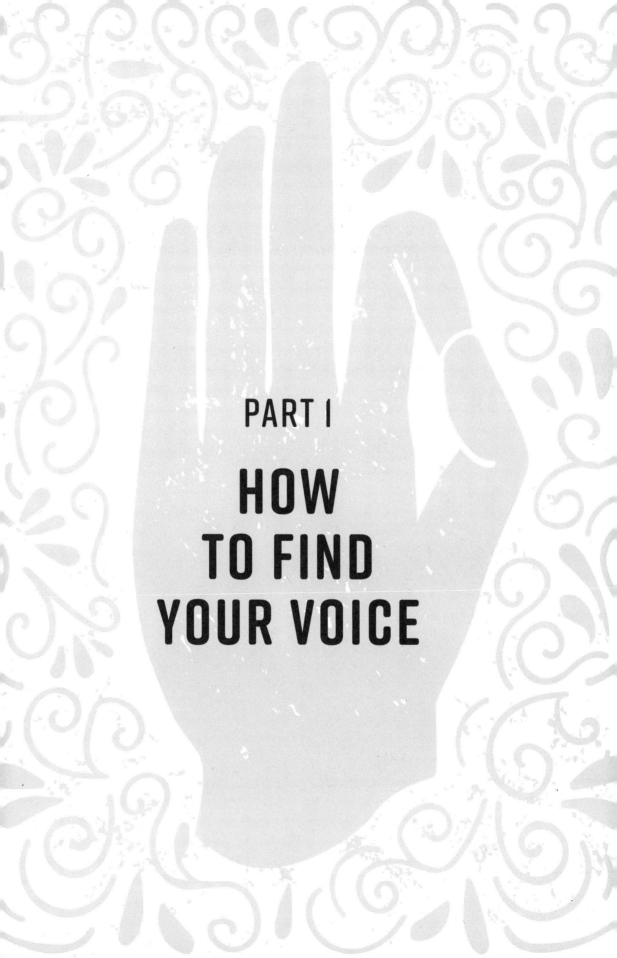

PART I

HOW TO FIND YOUR VOICE

1

WORDS ARE POWERFUL: THEMING MAKES YOUR CLASS

As leaders of yoga teacher trainings, we've got experience teaching the nuts and bolts of how to lead a helpful class. Once you've mastered those, the next challenge is adding meaning to your class by tying it to a theme or central message. This can be as elaborate as an explanation of yoga philosophy that is borne out in the sequences, or as simple as returning to the breath or remembering to relax.

A successful theme functions like a motif in classical music. It is gently but definitively introduced toward the beginning of the program, explored in various contexts over the course of the piece, and authoritatively revisited at the end. Perhaps at the beginning the central motif is played by one instrument. It is then taken up over the course of the piece by different instruments, each of which lend a unique tone, rhythm, and key to it. Finally, the entire ensemble joins in repeating the motif together.

Your class can carry a theme in a similar fashion. You'll introduce it using words in your opening comments, then students will consider the theme as they move through the class. Sometimes this means students will observe their embodied experience—how things feel in their bodies relative to the theme. Sometimes it means they will remember or repeat a word, phrase, or mantra tied to your theme. At the conclusion of class, you'll restate the theme again, and students can have time to reflect on its implications off the mat.

WHAT DOESN'T WORK

A successful theme is introduced early, referenced often, and reiterated at the end of class. Simply relating an undigested personal story, or reading a poem once and not referencing it further, does not deepen or enrich your students' experience. Be sure that you come back to your theme several times over the course of your class. While this may feel heavy-handed to you, remember that students process your words in the context of their own experience. If they are new, they may be focused mostly on the physical cues. If they are stressed, they may be focused on maintaining attention while their minds are tempted to ruminate or wander. If they are hard of hearing, they may not catch every word! What feels like too much repetition on your part is usually just right, since students will only really hear about half of what you say.

BUT WHY DOES THEMING MATTER?

You've picked up this book, we bet, because as a yoga student you have had at least one profound experience in a yoga class with a theme that affected you deeply. You already sense that saying beautiful, gently provocative, wise, and loving things while students move their bodies can shift them, transform them, and offer them relief from the daily existential suffering that typifies life for even the happiest of us. Theming matters not just because words are powerful, but also because you're presenting words and ideas to people when they are susceptible to listening to them—they are physically relaxed or physically challenged, mentally undistracted, and ready to receive. In the seat of the teacher, you're speaking to people when they are hungriest to hear instruction—not just on what to move or how to breathe, but also on how to *be*.

Theming in a yoga class matters a great deal. Offering your students a theme that allows them to have hope or peace or a renewed spirit is especially helpful in our present day, where politics, social unrest, and technology contribute to anxiety. Our colleague Leslie Kaminoff posted an important message on social media in the days following the 2016 election. He wrote, "All yoga educators: stress reduction is now the world's number-one growth industry. Let's do what we do best—stay centered and offer safe havens." His post resonated with us and reminded us that our job is to reduce the stress of our students. We can do that with thoughtful sequences, but we also need to offer nourishing class content.

Theming is one of the primary differences between a yoga practice and a fitness class. In a fitness class, students come to move, whether that's lifting weights, doing cardio step, cycling, or doing Pilates. Often, breath is cued in these classes, and excellent fitness instructors encourage self-care ("rest," "drink water") and self-awareness ("listen for the voice telling you that you can't do this—you can!"). But when students take a fitness class, they don't do so with the expectation that they will learn something—something philosophical, like a new life perspective—from the teacher.

But yoga nourishes the body *and* the soul; good theming makes that possible. When your students come to a yoga class, they want to feel better, and they also expect to learn something: they expect a side dish of philosophy with the main dish of yoga asana. They expect that as part of the practice of yoga, part of the experience of moving and breathing, there will also be a lesson or thought or advice about *being*.

To further this metaphor on eating, consider that doing yoga, like doing any sort of movement practice, is akin to eating a really healthy meal. It's enjoyable, in part because you know you're doing something good for yourself. But the best healthy meals are the ones that are not only good for you but are also delicious. The meals that are so delicious that you think of them later and want to make them again ("how could kale salad be that amazing?")—that's a yoga class with beautiful theming.

Theming also gets to the heart of ancient yoga, which began as a philosophical practice as the main with asana as the side dish. And while we're not purists and we love the ever-evolving exploration of yoga in the modern world, we also believe that yoga asana can't be divorced from its roots. Yoga is yoga today, and it's also the yoga of over two thousand years of philosophical thought. Yoga has always been used as a tool to help people with the daily challenges of living. Physical movement does a pretty good job of that on its own, but pairing movement with theming and wise words does it most fully. In offering your students wisdom on how to deal with the struggles of existence, you're connecting with the true history and purpose of yoga.

A FEW NOTES ON SPEAKING

We very much plan for this book to be a book on theming, not teaching. Although we might ask you to reflect on your preferences through journaling, we don't want to tell you how to cue or exactly what language to use. We assume that through training, emulation, and practice, you'll figure out the right fit for you as a teacher. But because this is a book literally about using your voice, we do want to mention a few key things about speaking well in a class setting.

1. Project your voice. When you have something to say, you have to speak loudly enough that your students can hear it. While you don't want to yell at your students, you do want them to hear you. When you speak in a class, speak to the person the farthest back—and imagine they have a hearing impairment. Speak up!

2. Allow silence. Full disclosure: both of us love to talk and probably still struggle with this ourselves. But learn from our challenge and allow silence to fill your yoga classroom. Allow silence, especially when students are in a restorative pose or holding a pose for a few breaths. Resist the urge to give every cue possible or to fill every second with your voice, lest your students tune it out.

3. Own your words. Whatever you say, say it with authority. Speak with certainty, and you'll feel more certain.

Aside from these three cardinal rules, you should explore to find your voice: clear and direct, warm and fuzzy, full of imagery, full of clear cues—you decide. But whatever your voice, speak up, speak with authority, and make room for silence.

2

WHAT DO OTHERS SAY?
THE ART OF EMULATION

The first step for you as a yoga teacher is learning what to say to get students safely into and out of the poses. But as a practitioner of yoga, you know that its power lies in the elements beyond the poses: the sense of connection, awareness, and union that comes from the complete practice. Now that you can cue a smart sequence of poses and usually keep right and left straight, how can you offer your students a full experience in your yoga class?

A seriously great place to start is to copy and borrow. Emulate your beloved mentors, teachers, writers, and colleagues! Go to classes and jot down the language your teacher uses that makes your heart feel lighter. Go home and journal on the intention that your teacher brought to class to open it more and see how it resonates further with you. Read a book that makes you genuinely feel happy and connected to humanity, and highlight every beautiful passage. New teachers may feel like this is not the place to begin, but we posit the opposite is true. As you find themes that resonate with your classes, emulation is an incredibly helpful starting point, not just because you'll find lovely tidbits that may stick with you forever, but also because you will very quickly notice what is *not* your voice or style.

Alexandra's toddler-aged daughter emulates everything Alexandra does to figure out her truth. She does this literally, parroting back things Alexandra says and the very way she says them, or trying on her shoes and jewelry. (So, of course, do Sage's teenaged daughters!) Sometimes things stick: she loves purple because Alexandra loves purple. But some things she tries and rejects. Toenail polish looked good on Alexandra's feet, but when—at her daughter's behest—she painted her toes to match Alexandra's, she was horrified, and immediately asked her to remove the garish color. We pay attention to the ways our children learn because it's the way human beings learn, toddlers, teens, or adults: we look to see what others do, and we try their way. If it's a good way, we keep doing it. If it's not, we don't.

BORROW FROM YOUR TEACHERS

When you begin teaching, copy the phrases, themes, and even nuances that your favorite teachers use. Try their ideas in your class. Say things the way they say things. Borrow their lessons and play with them on your home mat to see if they make sense. Try their words, and as they roll off your tongue, decide whether they feel like your truth too. Hear their words, then say their words. Sometimes we hear a beloved teacher say something that is so brave and unique and beautiful, we are moved in deeply emotional ways. We think about it later, for days. But then we try it ourselves, and it feels stale or flat or—worse—trite. Be willing to try on your teachers' words and intentions like you're open-mindedly trying on a variety of winter coats from a very full rack: tight-fitting and pleather, fluffy and warming, shellacked and waterproof, faux fur and glamorous. Try it all on, with an open mind and a playful attitude!

· · · · · · · · · **WORKBOOK EXERCISE: WHAT DO YOUR TEACHERS SAY?** · · · · · · · ·

As you begin to investigate the kind of language, metaphor, and tone that you would like to adopt, start with your favorite teachers. If you can find a video recording of a teacher you enjoy, sit and listen to the language. Perhaps you could audio record your teacher's class, with your teacher's permission and the clear parameter that this is solely for your own growth, not for distribution. Or, as soon as possible after class, make notes.

Pay special attention to:

- Pronouns. What pronouns does your teacher use, and in what amount? Is there more *I, you,* or *we?*

- Students don't hear everything you say. Sometimes they get into their own heads or are focused on breath. What phrases catch you? What does your teacher say that pulls you out of your head (in a helpful way)?

- What do you respond to emotionally? Do you find yourself smiling at some specific turn of phrase or aside? Why?

- Analogies, similes, and metaphors. Do these fall into a particular category, such as references to nature, the seasons, or current events? What makes these successful and appropriate for the class, level, or specific practice?

- Quotations, poems, chants, or music. How do these tie back into any expressed theme for class?

BORROW FROM TEXTS

If you want to inspire others, you have to read things that inspire you. Choose those inspirational texts from a place of authenticity too. If you feel your most balanced and present after reading something that others may consider banal, like a fashion magazine, then look for inspiration there! Look for quotes, lines, hopeful and honest perspectives, and heart-warming phrases. Look for themes for your practice. If you use social media, cull your threads so that you only see things that fill you up and offer ideas for your students to savor as they move and breathe.

BEING INFLUENCED VERSUS PLAGIARIZING: THE DIFFERENCE

We can't help but be shaped by our teachers and their language, voice, and intention. And we should be shaped by our knowledgeable mentors—otherwise why are we paying them for workshops and classes? Even after teaching for many years, we both still employ some phrases from our first teachers—those phrases work, and we've said them enough that they feel like our phrases now too. This is pretty common in yoga, and if you listen, you can hear it. Often you can trace the lineage of a teacher just by noticing the phrases they tend to use. Those cues or transitional phrases or Savasana language came from their teachers originally. So is it OK to take others' words and speak them as your own? You get to decide for yourself, of course, but here's where we land.

If you borrow language or a theme (or a sequence, while we're at it), we think it's a nice nod to the teacher to acknowledge to the students that this aspect of the yoga class did not originate with you. An easy way to do this is to say something like "One of my teachers always says …" or "My yoga mentor refers to this as …" or something similar. If you're inclined, say that teacher's name (especially if the teacher teaches in the area, and your students would enjoy his or her class too). By referencing or citing the originator of your words, you're acknowledging your own lineage as a teacher and sharing who and what has inspired you. You're assuming your place in the ancient tradition of yoga as a philosophy that was initially orally passed from teacher to student. And you're reminding your students that while you're leading the class, you're also a student too.

· · · · · · · · · · · · **WORKBOOK EXERCISE: READ FOR INSPIRATION** · · · · · · · · · · ·

Try this: grab a book or magazine that brings you joy to read, whether it's pulp mystery novels or *ESPN The Magazine*. Set a timer and read for five to ten minutes with the express purpose of looking for something that feels inspiring, that reminds you of the equally joyous and daunting task of being a human being on this earth, and that makes you feel slightly lighter or happier. Read for that, and when you find it, write about it here. Inspiration is everywhere.

3

AUTHENTICITY AND THE SEAT OF THE TEACHER

Authenticity is a buzzword that gets thrown around a lot in yoga. The best teachers are said to be the most authentic, and we think that's true in many ways. Or at least the opposite is true: inauthentic teachers are probably not going to be very popular. But isn't that the case for inauthentic people? We sniff them out, catching that something is slightly off. That off-ness is off-putting. In yoga, especially, where the practice of *svadhyaya* (self-study) is so important, someone who seems less than real is not going to be sought out.

CONFIDENCE AND AUTHENTICITY

When you feel nervous, insecure, afraid, or timid, it's hard to be authentic. Nervous energy and anxiety often read as inauthenticity, in part because they seem to transmit the idea that something is wrong. That's a frustrating reality for those of us who, by design of genetics, tend toward anxiety. The good news is that yoga gives us some tools for that, especially breath. The other good news is that most of this nervous energy and anxiety can be mitigated by thorough preparation.

Preparation begets confidence. When you've calmly planned your class sequence, including ways to expand or contract it for time; when you've lined up your music and collated your quotes; when you've set out the props each student will need and taken a moment to greet each student as they arrive—then you'll start class feeling confident. And if things go wrong, as they sometimes do, you'll have a plan to get back on track. Thinking through the potential pitfalls will help boost your confidence.

Thoughtful planning creates confidence, and your confidence makes students feel safe. If you seem to know what you're doing, even when you may not feel like you know what you're doing, your students feel that they are safe to trust you to lead them through movement and philosophy. This is important: when students feel safe, they let go more, and they get more out of the practice. Consider your most loved teachers: don't you trust them? And doesn't this trust translate for you into a deeper experience of movement and relaxation?

Authenticity from confidence can also be something that develops over time as you get a little more comfortable with your class and your students. When they come back time and again, revealing that they like and trust you, we bet you'll find it easier to be yourself more fully with them.

· · · · · · · · · · · **WORKBOOK EXERCISE: WHAT COULD GO WRONG?** · · · · · · · · · · ·

Write down how you want your students to feel at the end of your class. This could be *centered, balanced, happily fatigued, connected, ready for the day,* or whatever seems appropriate based on your class format and the time of day. This is your goal for the class.

Next, write out your road map for arriving at this destined goal. That can be a list of sequences, poses, a playlist, and quotes, as mentioned above, or it could be completing the templates you see in parts 2 and 3 of this book.

Now examine this plan with an eye for what might drive you off course. For example, your music app might be stuck on shuffle, you might have a pregnant student walk into a class that you have planned out to focus on prone backbends, or you might forget to include poses as you move through a sequence on the second side. Leave space under or alongside these potential road bumps.

Finally, consider how you can best get back on track or adapt with a detour should you encounter any of these obstacles. As you write down your strategies, note that some events are out of your control, and your best bet will be smiling, letting go of your plan, and finding the contentment in being in this new place. Other "disaster" events are not at all disastrous, and having planned how to handle them, you'll feel more confident walking into class. Write down your plans.

DO PEOPLE WANT YOU TO BE GENUINE? YES—AND NO

Let's start with the obvious: people want you to be genuinely you. They want to see your brand of humor, your compassion, and your values. When students return to your class, they do so because they've found something about you likeable, enjoyable, and sincere. They're there for yoga, but specifically *your* take on yoga. Cultivating honesty and authenticity will help you find students who will most love your classes. Being your true self will help you connect to your true students.

Sometimes, though, your genuine self is angry or heartbroken or broke. Sometimes your genuine self is feeling really down. This is where the words *genuine* and *authentic* can be confusing in the context of another important word: *professional*. You are a professional teacher, and your job is teaching yoga. That's the case whether it's a full-time job, a part-time job, or a hobby: when you agree to lead a class, professionalism comes with that responsibility. Ostensibly, the students who attend your class are paying you to lead them. Generally, that payment is in money, but it may also be a trade for services or it may even be a free class, in which case students are paying with their time and attention. If someone is paying you in any way to lead them through an inspiring yoga practice, there is definitely room for your authentic self. But you have to be sure that your authentic self doesn't detract from the experience you're trying to create.

Here's what we mean. Imagine you show up for a massage ready to be quiet and let your stresses melt away, and in need of deep tissue work for tight quads. You go to a massage therapist you really like and that you've been to before, but when you arrive, he is obviously distracted and seems sad. You ask, politely, if everything is OK, and he tells you he's going through a significant breakup. Because he seems in need of care, and because you truly like this person, you ask questions and the two of you talk about his heartbreak through the massage. Because you are empathetic, you don't remind him that your quads are really tight when he seems to have forgotten the deep-tissue work you need— he is distracted for a good reason: his heart is broken! At the end of the massage, he thanks you for being so supportive and kind. And you leave feeling kind for listening to him, but having given a lot of money and a lot of time for a service that didn't quite meet what you needed. Would you go back? Would you feel a little bummed out to have spent your money and time on a massage that wasn't great and that actually required you to expend energy?

As a teacher, don't take up so much space that your students can't relax or release or let go. Don't share so much of your sadness or frustration or your troubles that your students feel the need to support you or lift you up. Don't ask your students to give to you emotionally when part of your job as a professional yoga teacher is to give time and energy to your students. It is not an equal exchange of energy. Your students are not your friends. We talk more in chapter 6 about what to do when you feel like you have very little to give, and there are certainly ways to teach a good class when you're in that empty-well place. But we don't think taking energy from your students is very professional, even if it is genuine sometimes. So if you feel like you have to choose between the two things, genuine emotion or professionalism, choose the latter. Or get a sub.

YOGA VOICE AND IDENTITY

We like when a teacher's voice in the classroom is not so dissimilar to what it would be in the grocery store. Having a "yoga teacher voice" that is radically different from your own daily voice doesn't resonate as authentic. We make certain changes when we step into a classroom—we are more considerate of our words, we're more professional, and our language might be more conceptual—but ultimately we are ourselves. Consider that if your "yoga voice" were so radically different from your own voice, you would have to be choreographing a class, thinking of clever things to say, and also acting—a triple load of effort that is not only unnecessary, it's also inauthentic.

Investigate your natural voice. What do you sound like in casual everyday conversation? Consider too what you enjoy hearing in a yoga class. What soothes you and puts you in the moment? In looking at your natural voice and your idealized voice, we hope that you find what we imagine is true: your ideal yoga voice is just another version of your natural voice—albeit one, perhaps, with more pauses or clearer pronunciation or stronger projection.

········· WORKBOOK EXERCISE: SPEAKING OF AUTHENTICITY ... ·········

Naturally, we all adopt slightly different personas based on the situation. But your unique, authentic voice is the bedrock on which each of these variations rests. Take some time to journal in exploration of what makes your voice unique and authentic. Are you naturally quiet or loud? A person of few words, or a chatterbox? Are you calm or animated? When you are at ease with friends and family, what does your voice sound like? What role do you play in your friend group? Do you use colorful language or even—*gasp!*—curse sometimes, and if so, in which situations?

Next, write a little about what you enjoy as the "ideal yoga teacher voice." Is it well projected? Patient? Are there periods of silence between the sentences, or does your teacher fill the space? Is there humor? Is the ideal yoga teacher voice monotone or dynamic? There is not one right answer to these questions. Consider what *you* enjoy hearing in classes you take.

Finally, write about the intersection between your authentic voice and the ideal yoga teacher voice you envision. In what ways does your authentic voice—your natural way of relating and speaking—already connect to the idealized yoga voice you imagine?

VULNERABILITY AND AUTHENTICITY

As we've already noted, openness and authenticity tend to resonate with students. They tend to resonate with everyone, actually, but are particularly prized in a yoga setting, where being present is something most students and teachers are actively working on. As part of the practice of yoga, we're trying to see others wholly, to be in the moment, and to be ourselves most truly.

Being authentic means that you show up to teach as your professional and honest self, and you hope that self resonates with others. We're saying this rather casually, but in reality it can be terrifying. So let's not make light of it: when you feel that you are truly yourself and teaching from a place of authenticity, but in the following weeks none of the same students return to your class—well, it can feel pretty damn soul- (and wallet-) crushing. Now, please keep in mind that most of the time, if a student doesn't return to your class, it has nothing to do with you. Students show up—or not—for their practice for so many different reasons, and we suspect that it rarely truly has to do with the teacher. Still, being authentic requires deep bravery in the face of inevitable rejection. That's definitely a part of being human, and it's definitely a part of being a yoga teacher. You will show up as yourself, and some people will not like the way you teach, or your voice, or your lesson, or your sequence, or even just you. Oh, well.

Experiencing rejection means that you are pushing your own boundaries of personal comfort. It means you are challenging yourself to do risky things. It means you are putting yourself out there. Still, because rejection is part of being a yoga teacher, being just you—you as you are—can feel deeply vulnerable. There's not much to be done about it, except to acknowledge it, sit with it, and meditate on it with the hope of accepting it as an inevitable part of the path you have chosen.

One thing we want to make clear, though, is that while being authentic can *feel* vulnerable, authenticity and vulnerability are not the same thing. Here's what we mean: we all have things that make us feel embarrassed, small, vulnerable. Maybe you've recently gone through a divorce or breakup. Maybe you have a tough family background. Maybe you struggle with depression or anger. All of these things are perfectly normal, of course, and nothing to be ashamed of. They're good things to discuss with trusted friends, loved ones, and well-trained therapists.

· · · · · · · · · **WORKBOOK EXERCISE: THE EXPERIENCE OF REJECTION** · · · · · · · ·

Imagine a scenario where you have felt rejected. It doesn't have to be connected to yoga, but it could be, if you have experienced a similar scenario to the one we described above: students coming to your class but not returning, for instance. First, write a little (as descriptively as possible) about how rejection *feels*. Does it feel hot? Does it feel sharp? What does the experience of rejection feel like in your body? Next, write about what you learned, if anything, from this experience of rejection. Did you learn about things you want to do differently? Did you learn that rejection is normal? Finally, write a little about how this sentence makes you feel: All successful people experience rejection on the path to success.

But you are not required under any circumstances to sit on your mat and share your vulnerabilities or insecurities with your class. That's not remotely a part of authenticity. You don't have to speak from that place, and you don't have to share your personal life with your students beyond professional basics. Authenticity—being yourself, speaking the way you speak, being professional and polite as part of your job—is not the same as opening yourself up in ways that are uncomfortable and unnecessarily vulnerable.

That's not to say that you can't *ever* share openly about your own life crises in class. We know some very skilled yoga teachers who like to be open and teach from a personal place. They comfortably share the things they are currently and personally working on, and they do so in a way that is beneficial for their students, through sharing lessons, yoga philosophy, and helpful mantras that they've found useful. They balance sharing and authentic teaching, and they do so because that's what feels right for them. If that *is* your authentic way of being, go for it! But please don't feel that if you tend to be a private person that anything needs to change. You do not need to reveal anything more than you want to. And if you do like to personally share, keep the concept of oversharing in your mind too. If you are sharing so much or so emotionally that your students feel that they have to attend to you, you may not know it immediately. But we suspect you'll realize it when they don't return to your class. Students are coming to enjoy an experience of breath, movement, and philosophy, not to give empathy and energy to you.

When you look at how authenticity and vulnerability play a role in your teaching, recognize that it can *feel* vulnerable to be authentic because there is always the possibility of rejection, which hurts. But that's part of this job. You are required—by virtue of being a yoga teacher—to show up authentically and do your best to give energy to your students. But authenticity is not vulnerability, and you aren't required to share your vulnerabilities with anyone you don't know well, love and trust deeply, or pay for advice.

4

PRACTICE YOUR WORDS UNTIL YOU BELIEVE THEM

The hardest part of theming well is that you may be talking about philosophical concepts, ideas, or lessons that you don't have spaces in the "real world" to discuss—so make those spaces. If your yoga themes exist only in a yoga studio, they'll never seem authentic to you or your students. You have to choose themes that interest you, surprise you, intrigue you, or excite you. These themes have to be ones that feel like guideposts in your life, so much so that you want to bring them into everyday conversation, whether with your partner, friends, or checkout clerk (unlikely, we admit, but not impossible). All of this sharing and discussion gives you ample opportunity to practice your theme. The more you talk about the themes that resonate with you, the more these themes feel authentically yours. You have to practice your ideas and your words until they feel like they're yours—until you believe them.

WRITE IT

When you happen upon a theme that speaks to you, whether it's yoga philosophy, poetry, a quote, personal observation, or a song lyric, the first thing to do is write it down. Ideally, you should be writing your immediate tidbits of inspiration in one place, like this book! Chapter 16 is a great place to jot down ideas that you want to flesh out later. Collect ideas like a magpie collecting shiny objects. Everything that sparkles should be gathered! In college, Alexandra was lucky enough to study under American poets David Kirby and Barbara Hamby, whose primary advice was to write everything down—everything that strikes you can be art. That was their take, and it's ours too. In becoming good at theming, you have to collect ideas that resonate.

Not only should you collect ideas and write them down, though, you should also write *about* them. Sometimes freewriting can help you better determine what's at the heart of the idea for you—what's important about it? We've given you a lot of directed journal prompts in this book, but sometimes the most revealing writing sessions are the ones that are freestyle and undirected. When an idea strikes you as a possible theme, put your pen to paper (or your hands to keyboard or your thumbs to your phone) and dash off a little bit about why you like it. Why does it speak to you?

· · · · · · · · · · · · · · · **WORKBOOK EXERCISE: FREEWRITE!** · · · · · · · · · · · · · · ·

Choose an idea that has been on the periphery of your mind for a while. Maybe you haven't even written the idea down yet. Jot it here, even if it's only half-formed, and spend three to five minutes freewriting. You may even want to time yourself. Write, investigating your thoughts and feelings about the idea, and see what bubbles up. If you get stuck, keep writing, even if it's "I'm stuck, I'm stuck, I'm stuck."

DISCUSS IT

As you have new ideas and themes marinating, it's useful to bring those ideas into conversations with your friends and loved ones. You can be candid about what you're doing: tell them, "Hey, I just read this tidbit of yoga philosophy, and it really clicks," and then share it. See what they say; consider how they react. Likely, they'll have a comment or observation that will deepen your experience of the theme. Bring your potential themes into casual everyday conversation; we promise that once you've done this, bringing those same themes to your yoga class will feel so much more natural.

For some of us, discussing and conversing on ideas and themes is an important part of knowing what we really think—saying something out loud helps us hear it as true. Discussing a yoga theme, talking about it, and even debating its merits with a friend or partner can help you develop the theme, understand it, and identify the aspects that seem the most important to stress in a class with your students.

PROCLAIM IT

If you use social media, you have an easy outlet right there: share what inspires you and watch how others respond. Be sure to credit your original source. Consider adding a follow-up question to your quote, so that you elicit a discussion from your followers. This can lead to a productive give-and-take that deepens your connection to and understanding of the quote or idea, which in turn can help you develop it into a meaningful theme for class. And bonus: as your yoga students begin to follow you in an online capacity, they'll get to hear your prominent themes multiple times. That's great for them: when a theme really resonates, they'll be exposed to it online *and* in your yoga class, and the power of the words or ideas will grow stronger because of that.

LISTEN AND FEEL FOR WHAT DOESN'T STICK

Practice your words, yes. But also be OK with trying a theme and then pitching it into the garbage directly after your class. Sometimes words seem to flow easily and float around the yoga room, but other times it feels like they fall from your mouth and thud to the floor, clumsy, useless. That's good—just like you need to appreciate the times you fall out of a balance pose in order to learn to find the sweet spot in it, you also have to practice your language, tone, and expressions so that you can hit your mark most of the time.

But please know: often it's the classes that we feel were most underwhelming that land most deeply with our students. And often it's the students who leave class without a glance to the teacher who write emails later saying, "That was just what I needed to hear." Don't beat yourself up when you feel like you have an off day. It may have actually been exactly what your students needed.

THEMING IS A LOT OF WORK!

We figure you might be thinking this right now, so we want to address it: yes, theming can be a lot of work. But remember that in this book, we give you fifty-four completed themes that you can work with. Remember also that while we hope you'll create another fifty-four or more on your own, so you have a huge toolkit of themes to work from, we bet you'll find that you come back to the same twenty or so themes again and again. With that idea in mind, you'll see that theming is a lot of work at first, but it gets easier once you've identified themes that you love to talk about. After that, it's just a matter of occasionally updating or refreshing themes when things start to feel stale.

5

REPETITION IS COMFORTABLE (AND STUDENTS WANT TO BE COMFORTABLE)

A good yoga class contains the right balance of consistency and variety. The basic structure—centering, warmups, poses, Savasana, closing—must be the same week to week, or students will never learn the fundamentals. The particulars of what happens in class, though, must change relative to the students' experience and expectations, so that students can remain challenged and engaged. With too much consistency, there's no growth; with too much variety, there's no stability.

This is true not only for the sequence of poses you teach, but also for the words you use. If there's a new and disparate lesson each week that doesn't reference what has come before, students won't connect with the basics of yoga philosophy. On the other hand, if you make the same point week in and week out, students may get bored and definitely will miss out on the wide range of life lessons yoga themes and philosophy can offer.

REPETITION HELPS

The joke goes: "What are the three most important keys to learning?" "Repetition, repetition, repetition."

You are the only one who has ever been in every class you've taught. And you are the only one who has ever heard every single word you've ever said. While you may have heard the words a million times, your students have not. They cherish the repetition—it creates consistency for them. Not only do your students learn through repetition, they may need to hear something over and over and over until it finally lands. Once it has landed, they are still happy to hear it again, as returning to the same idea over and over both feels reassuring—like returning to the same favorite vacation spot—and gives students a chance to connect more deeply and to see different subtleties each time.

There will be certain phrases and cues you repeat dozens of times per class. Chief among them: "Breathe." Sage's go-to cue works well with populations of athletes, type A's, and just about anyone: "Where could you do less?" This can run through various permeations: "Where could you do less and achieve the same results?" "Where could you do less and feel better?" "Where could you do less and catch yourself creating more work than needed?" Alexandra loves "Let your body breathe" as a way to cue relaxation at the start or end of a practice. It's a sweet reminder to let your mind slow down and allow your body to just be and breathe. She says this phrase most classes, but also modifies it for challenging poses: "Can you let your body breathe here?" or "Even as we hold this for a few more moments, can you soften and breathe?"

Listen to your own most-repeated phrases. You'll find in them the germ of your top ten themes. If you aren't sure what your go-to words and phrases are, record your class. You'll very quickly notice the things you repeat that add value, like "Breathe" or "Do less" or "Soften your jaw and face," as well as filler words and phrases like "um," "and now, from here, we're going to," or any other personal tics you might like to drop.

· · · · · · · · · · **WORKBOOK EXERCISE: REPETITION WITH VARIATION** · · · · · · · · ·

Since yoga studios sit empty for part of the afternoon, Carolina Yoga Company used to rent space to Keith, a working actor who wanted a neutral studio for practice. He warned us not to be alarmed if we overheard part of his warm-up, which involved repeating "How dare you?" at a variety of volumes, in a variety of tones, as a variety of characters. (Unfortunately, we never did get to hear Keith do this!)

Once you are clear on your most useful phrases to repeat, find ways to vary them so that each one is unique, just like Keith saying, "How dare you?" In this journal space, start by making a list of your most-used yoga teaching and cuing phrases. Next, write out a few variations on the same phrase. After that, be sure also to practice saying them out loud with inflection that shades their meaning. You'll learn the most if you are brave enough to record yourself doing this, and to play it back with a friendly ear and an open mind.

···· TOO MUCH REPETITION DEADENS ····

As you've likely noticed, each radio station has a self-identifying phrase to be repeated hourly as station identification to comply with US Federal Communications Commission regulations. Announcers quickly learn exactly how long their station identification takes—it's often ten seconds or less—and how quickly they can say it if they are running low on time. The challenge, as Sage learned in her six years of announcing on public radio, is to say the station identification in a human tone, instead of repeating it in a monotone like a robot.

Think of flight attendants rattling off the safety instructions like automatons. They're bored, the passengers are bored, and the message is lost in the delivery. That's a shame, as it's potentially life-or-death information. Compare this with the flight instructions you hear on a Southwest Airlines flight. The attendants each bring their own personality to the spiel, there's usually some surprising or silly component, and consequently the passengers pay attention.

The same thing is true of yoga teachers. We can find ourselves depending on stock phrases ("The light in me honors the light in you") delivered in the same robotic tone, class in and class out. Again, if you aren't sure whether you do this, audio or video record your class, and you'll very quickly hear it. Workshop these phrases to develop a more interesting and engaging class.

That's not to say that if you use a phrase like "The light in me honors the light in you" that it's necessarily rote or devoid of meaning. It has a lot to do with whether you feel it or infuse it with meaning—and whether or not the phrase really matters to you when you say it.

· · · · · · · · · · **WORKSHOP EXERCISE: ENLIVEN YOUR BOILERPLATE** · · · · · · · · · ·

Write down your go-to beginning-of-class and end-of-class blurbs, whether they are a welcome you always deliver or the closing words you find yourself rushing through at the end of class. You'll likely find this is an easy task, since you say the same words in the same order every time.

Now find at least three different ways to convey the information, so that the message remains the same but the presentation varies. Once you've written them down, repeat them until they feel comfortable and familiar, while still fresh. Repeat this exercise every six or twelve months, so that you don't fall into the stale rut in the future.

· ·

REPETITION OF THEMES THROUGH THE YEAR

By the end of this book, you'll have read through more than enough themes to carry you through a whole year of weekly classes—and if you create another fifty-four or more, there's another year covered! But you don't really need to introduce a brand-new theme every week. In fact, that might skew your offering too far into variety and away from consistency.

You'll likely instead find that certain themes resonate best with you and with your students. Those are the ones you'll want to keep in the heavy rotation across the calendar year. There are others that are seasonally appropriate, and yet others that might feel germane because of something happening personally, locally, or globally.

Just as you shouldn't fear repetition in your language, don't worry about repeating themes year in and year out. As long as you bring something fresh to them (and you will because *you* change and grow every year), your students will not only appreciate but actively crave revisiting themes.

6

FINDING INSPIRATION— AND WHAT TO DO WHEN YOU'RE NOT INSPIRED

No one wakes up every day with a full-throttle smile, grateful, and prancing out of bed like a Disney-movie animal sidekick. You probably do know people like that, but rest assured, we're not them. Yoga teachers and practitioners are human, and that means waking up cranky sometimes, or being stressed by work or family, or not getting enough sleep. Let us say that again: yoga teachers are human. Even the most loved gurus have an off day. And a common joke in yoga teacher circles is that yoga teachers might actually tend toward the moody as they are often the *most* intensely emotional or type-A people: we've found ourselves drawn to yoga as a way to regulate that emotional intensity.

Some days, you may find yourself rolling out your mat, ready to lead or practice yoga from a serene place of equanimity. Teaching and doing yoga after a night of good sleep, a harmonious week, and from a place of peace is, of course, a bit easier. And while the point of a yoga practice is to arrive at that peace, it's unrealistic to imagine that you'll start from there every practice, especially as the teacher. When you're in an inspirational rut, it's useful to have some tools for your theming. In this chapter, we'll offer you a few exercises for finding inspiration and a few tips for staying inspired. But we'll also offer you the most important tool of all: the ability to let yourself off the hook when you just feel like you have nothing to say to inspire others—or yourself. That's part of the practice of yoga too, and it's OK to be an exhausted and cranky teacher sometimes—we promise, you can still teach a good class! Say it with us now: yoga teachers are human.

FINDING INSPIRATION

When you feel stuck, but not so stuck that you're unable to find *something* that inspires you, explore this section. Maybe you feel like your themes in class have grown too lengthy or become a word salad. Maybe you feel like you've been saying the same things to yourself or your students again and again. When you've worked your way through the length of this book, you'll have 108 or more complete themes to come back to. But until then, here are some exercises that can help bring out your creative, inspired self.

WORKBOOK EXERCISE: GRATITUDE LISTS

Writing down a list of things that you're grateful for is a standard prompt in self-help books, therapy work, and in the growing focus on daily practices that can help you be happier. There's a reason that gratitude lists are everywhere: they work. Here are two approaches to gratitude lists that can help you find a new theme or bit of inspiration for your practice or class.

LIST 1

Make a list of the reasons you're most grateful for your yoga practice. Get as silly and specific as you can. (When Alexandra made this list, her first item was "I get to wear yoga pants every single day.") If you want, start with this question: What makes you happiest about finding yoga?

Take a few minutes resting in a restorative pose (like Supported Fish Pose or your favorite shape) to meditate on the answer. And then write. If you've been practicing yoga for a while, this list may help you connect with the roots of your practice.

LIST 2

Make a list of reasons you feel grateful *today*. Those ideas don't have to be centered on something that's specifically happening now, but may hark back to circumstances that allowed you to arrive where you are in life now. (Something like "I'm grateful I moved to this state after college, so I get to experience the beautiful fall season every year" works nicely.) If you're writing from a place of unhappiness or deep frustration, start very small: find gratitude for your breath, your quiet space, your cup of tea. Notice the little bits of peace that exist around you.

· · · · · · · · · · · **WORKBOOK EXERCISE: NAME YOUR EMOTIONS** · · · · · · · · · · ·

Research shows that naming your emotions as clearly and specifically as you can helps you process them and understand them better, according to Tony Schwartz in "The Importance of Naming Your Emotions" (*New York Times,* June 3, 2016). Getting awareness that you're being affected by your emotions and then striving to specify what, exactly, those emotions are can help you assimilate them, rather than be driven by them. Notice how you're feeling today and see what you can say about it. Start from a general emotion: *I'm feeling sad.* But then get to the heart of it, as precisely as you can. Here's an example: *I'm feeling deep ennui over the passage of time; fall weather always does that to me! I'm also feeling a sense of grim despair over the recent political news—it's hard to stay hopeful when there is nonstop crazy news coming from our social leaders. Finally, I'm feeling tired: I didn't sleep well last night, and I'm sure that a lack of sleep is affecting my view of the world and life today.*

·············· WORKBOOK EXERCISE: UNEXPECTED JOY ··············

Cataloging each day's unexpected joys (#ujoy) is Sage's useful daily tool for noticing the potential for happiness that exists all around. You'll see this idea appear later in our sample themes. But it also works as a way to find inspiration. The first step is to pay attention to what's happening around you. The second step is to look for the good in unexpected places—an interaction with a stranger, a tree that seems to have a face, any minor but joyous surprise. Once you tune in to unexpected joy, you'll begin to see it more and more frequently. List a few things that have been a welcome, unforeseen surprise for you lately.

· ·

················ **WORKBOOK EXERCISE: YOUR BIG LESSONS** ··············

When you look at your life in hindsight, you probably notice the stories that you tell and retell, the choices you made that seem to have mattered the most profoundly, and the lessons you feel were hard-won. Those lessons are the big themes of your life, and when you identify them, you'll always have an authentic, personal theme to come back to and speak from. It may be that sharing the deeply personal aspect of this life theme is *too* personal to share with a class—and that's totally reasonable. Still, identifying the themes and lessons that have shaped you will allow you to feel like an expert on these topics. And it's much easier to teach, lead, and practice from a place of expertise and authenticity.

Start by writing a little about each of these questions: What is the biggest, hardest choice you made in your life, and why did you make it? What did you learn from making this choice? What has been your greatest loss and your greatest gain so far?

STAYING FRESH

When you do find yourself in those life or inspiration ruts, using a workbook exercise to write your way out of it is a good approach. But it's also useful to check in with your life practices. Are you taking care of yourself? Are you actively open to and searching for inspiration?

Self-Care

The single most important way to stay ready to teach yoga and ready to practice is to engage in self-care. Your free time and your budget can help you define self-care for yourself, but at the very least, it is necessary that you have the space to get enough sleep, the openness in your week to have at least one day off, and the opportunity (and self-love!) to give to yourself in some gently indulgent way, whether that is a home pedicure, sleeping in, attending a restorative yoga class, or getting a massage. It is not possible to give to others (which is pretty much the job, if you teach yoga) from an empty well. Define for yourself what makes you feel filled up, taken care of, rested, safe, and well. And then prioritize those things in your week. Self-care is health care. It is not optional.

Take Classes (with an Open Mind!)

If you are a dedicated home practitioner, you might find yourself always drawn to your own mat and the solitude of your own space. But getting to a class with a popular or a fresh teacher may help you find a new approach, a new perspective, or a wonderful theme that resonates. If possible, take at least one studio yoga class each week. And even if you have teachers that you're drawn to and love, challenge yourself to vary your class attendance and try new teachers and classes, ever widening your perspective and freshening the messages you're receiving. If you're a teacher, up the challenge even more: *go to classes without mentally critiquing them.* This can be especially hard if you're newly graduated from yoga teacher training, which often has built-in time for self-critique and group teaching feedback. Try to quiet the voices in your head that notice a teacher's verbal tics or that always want to guess the next part of the sequence before it arrives. Just focus on moving your body and listening to the teacher—come to class open and hungry to be inspired, and you will be.

Read, Read, Read

We'll say it again: whether it's fiction, yoga philosophy, or the *New York Times,* read a little every day, seeking inspirational ideas, quotes, and perspectives. Find a way to save the things that you love so you can easily find them again. Technology makes this pretty easy. Read things that make you feel joyful, curious, hopeful, and open. And while we're at it: consider limiting articles or books that do the opposite. Nothing shuts down inspiration as quickly as despair, and the modern twenty-four-hour news cycle is an ever-producing despair machine. Limit your consumption!

WHAT TO DO WHEN YOU'RE NOT INSPIRED

No matter how much self-care you practice, how much sleep you get, and how many Mary Oliver poems you read, you will have some days that you just don't have anything uplifting or helpful to say. Rest assured that that's just fine, and you can come to the seat of the teacher with an empty well and still teach a beautiful class. Here's how.

Have a Back-Pocket Theme

Have a go-to theme that is broad enough to always be authentic and helpful enough that your students will always resonate. You'll find some of these in our sample themes chapter, but you probably already have your own, even if you don't realize it. Alexandra comes back to "This is what's happening now" as a class theme repeatedly, and it's always fresh and inspired, since it always encourages students (and Alexandra) to notice the *now.* Sage's go-to is finding the balance between effort and ease, making and letting, stress and rest, as it always seems to land with students, whether the class is vigorous or very gentle.

Just Breathe

If you have nothing to say to yourself or your students, focus on breath. This is a profound practice that is always helpful for students. If you're comfortable teaching a variety of *pranayama* practices, theme your class around trying various breaths (bee breath, alternate-nostril breathing, Lion's Breath, three-part breath, etc.) in various poses or parts of the practice. This focus on breath is easy to teach when you feel like you have less to say. And it doesn't even have to be that complicated: you don't have to teach various approaches to breathing; you can simply lead students (and yourself!) back to the breath again and again. Theme complete.

Alexandra attended a Yoga and Positive Psychology workshop with our beloved teacher Michael Johnson, and she asked him how yoga teachers should handle teaching from a dark place: What do we do as teachers when we arrive on our mats from a completely shitty day? How do we come up with a theme? How do we talk authentically about peace or presence when we feel neither peaceful nor present? What do we say? His response released her from ever scrambling again. "Don't try," he said. "Just gently lead your students through the poses and remind them to breathe." He reminded her that when that's all she has to give, that *is* her authentic theme. Yes, this book is about theming, and we do believe that the best yoga classes and practices have a clear intention. But when you have nothing to give, the best thing to do is scale back and give what you can: movement and breath. Sometimes those essential elements of yoga are theme enough.

While we were drafting this book, Sage was visiting her mother-in-law when she awoke to flames at 2 a.m. Monday morning and had to rouse the whole household to evacuate while the house burned down. She wrote Alexandra at 3 a.m. asking her to sub her 6 p.m. class, but when her mother-in-law insisted Sage and her family head home, she wound up teaching the class herself. Did she mention the fire to her students? Of course, in case she seemed extra tired or flubbed "right" and "left." Did she make a theme out of the fire? No, it was too fresh and unprocessed. Some day that theme will come; on this day, teaching movement and breath in the service of connection was enough, and it felt good to her to work in service to her students instead of focusing on her own traumatic experience.

Sometimes life circumstances and news render even the most carefully planned theme inadequate. Sage has had to teach the day of and the day after the Sandy Hook, Pulse Nightclub, and Las Vegas mass shootings, when anything she could say felt puny in the face of such tragedy. The most challenging experience of her decade and a half of teaching yoga was in a regular private lesson she gives to a couple and their best friend, who showed up on the mat for their regular practice two days after her husband died. What could she say to their grief? "Thanks for showing during such a hard time and having faith in this practice. We're here; let's breathe."

PART 2

FIFTY-FOUR COMPLETE THEMES

In this part of the book, we offer our template for theming classes along with fifty-four complete themes. We want to model the idea of flexibility by offering a template with lots of options—and in some themes, making wise choices about which aspects of the template to use.

We created fifty-four themes for two reasons. First, having fifty-four themes gives you more than a theme a week for a year. If you're in a rut or you're in the process of developing your own voice and themes, you have a lot to draw from here. Next, fifty-four is half of 108, a number that is venerated in yoga. (It's considered sacred for several reasons, and there is much open to interpretation.) We liked the idea that the number of themes we created were in themselves thematic and connected to the wisdom and traditions of yoga.

As you use these themes, you can choose to use our exact words, if you try them on for size and they fit. You can also use these templates as a rough guide of what it looks like to intertwine a theme through your class. You can pick and choose the phrases or ideas that most resonate from each theme. These templates still give you choice and room for creativity and interpretation. For instance, we have often included a song or two that connects to a specific theme to us. You could create a yoga playlist building from these songs. (Or ignore them: we don't play music in all our classes.) For some themes, we included chants, if you like to add that element into your classes. For some themes, we have included poems, since we've found that students often enjoy having a literary connection to the philosophy we're presenting (and we both studied literature, so we appreciate that too). But pick and choose and find the parts that resonate. As you use these themes, write down other ideas that come to you or mark the words that flow especially well for you. Your classes will appreciate your dedication to moving their practice beyond the poses.

7

THE BASICS OF YOGA PHILOSOPHY: TEACHING THE *YAMAS* AND *NIYAMAS*

AHIMSA

Write a Little about Your Theme and Why It Speaks to You

The first *yama* (ethical commandment) is *ahimsa*. *Ahimsa*, which translates to "nonviolence" or "nonharming," is at the heart of practicing yoga. Your practice on the mat should be about love, not harm, for yourself; your practice off the mat can continue that love toward yourself and others. *Ahimsa* is a reminder that all actions can come from a place of love. It's a reminder that at the heart of yoga is love.

Chants, Quotes, Mantras, Poems, or Songs That Connect

First, do no harm.

"To curb [violence] what is most needed is freedom from fear." —B. K. S. Iyengar, *Light on Yoga*

"Bomb the World" by Michael Franti

"Peace Train" by Cat Stevens

Poses That Work with Your Theme

Seated meditation and Supine meditation. But also, cuing more challenging poses (like Full Wheel or Eight-Angle Pose) with a reminder to do them from a place of *ahimsa* can be helpful for students who like challenge but might appreciate the reminder to move with love at the heart of the challenge.

Distill Your Theme to a Short Sentence or Intention

Move with love.

Phrases or Sentences to Employ in These Parts of Your Class

OPENING	DURING MOVEMENTS
The most important ethical precept is this: nonviolence. And while you are probably not an overtly violent person (we hope not!), Iyengar reminds us that "violence is a state of mind." Every pose that we do today can be done from a place of harming or nonharming. Allow yourself to flow with love, not force.	At the heart of every pose, breath, and word can be *ahimsa*. Move with love. As you enter this pose, can you do so peacefully? As you try this next pose, know that those around you are trying it too—you're in a community of support, all of us moving with love.
DURING PAUSES	**CLOSING**
Let your breath slow, and feel your heart rate calm. Here we are in peace, breathing. Peace and love are the opposite of violence, harm, and fear. Feel this peace now.	Can you take this feeling of love and peace with you off the mat? Can you move with nonviolence when you're cut off in traffic or when you're coming home to cranky children? Nonviolence is a state of mind, and the true practice of yoga happens off the mat, not on it. Move with love.

Anything Else

Every yoga philosopher has a slightly different approach to *ahimsa,* and it shows up in Buddhism too. It's worth continuing to explore this theme by reading about it more.

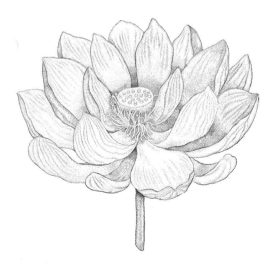

SATYA

Write a Little about Your Theme and Why It Speaks to You

The second of the *yamas, satya,* means "truth." In our quest to become authentic yogis, is there any place for dishonesty, which is fundamentally inauthentic? How can we find our own truth if we don't behave truthfully with others? As B. K. S. Iyengar teaches it, to be dishonest means we're out of harmony with the world. T. K. V. Desikachar complicates it so nicely, though, by reminding us that "*Satya* should never come into conflict with our efforts to behave with *ahimsa.*" Essentially, if speaking truthfully hurts others, then hold your tongue. This is a helpful reminder that the modern world is a complicated place, and we have to do our best to act out of love and honesty—and also acknowledge that they do sometimes contradict each other.

At the heart of being honest, though, is a desire to be honest *with ourselves*: that's why the idea of "finding your truth" or "speaking your truth" is such a common part of modern-day yoga. Being honest in that sense takes a lot of bravery! First, you have to practice enough *svadhyaya* to know what you really believe. Then, you have to be willing to say what you think and feel, even if that's at odds with what others think or feel. That's *satya* in its most refined form: living your truth.

Chants, Quotes, Mantras, Poems, or Songs That Connect

Om Kriyam Namah ("My actions are aligned with the universe.")

"There is no greater agony than bearing an untold story inside you." —Zora Neale Hurston, *Dust Tracks on a Road*

"True mind is our real self." —Thich Nhat Hanh, *The Miracle of Mindfulness*

Poses That Work with Your Theme

Heart-opening poses work great with themes about personal truth: Camel, Bow, Full Wheel, and the like. Lion's Breath, where you stick out your tongue as you exhale, can underline the idea of letting your voice flow. Meditation is a good option too.

Distill Your Theme to a Short Sentence or Intention

What is your personal truth?

Listen deeply: what do you hear?

Phrases or Sentences to Employ in These Parts of Your Class

OPENING

We hear a lot about "finding your truth" in our modern culture, but what does this mean? And how do we "find" truth? In reality, finding your truth is about listening better to what you're already saying to yourself. Your innate wisdom is there. The answers are inside. There's no finding to be done: all you have to do is listen. Yoga and meditation give us the space and silence to hear, to listen to what is already there.

DURING MOVEMENTS

Arrive in the pose.

Radiate from the pose.

Find yourself in this pose.

Move with integrity.

Here are options: practice the pose that aligns with what's right for you.

DURING PAUSES

What do you hear here, when you listen?

Pause in this in-between space and hear your heartbeat, hear your inner self.

What does your body tell you now?

CLOSING

In this space of silence before you move into the world, listen again to your deepest voice. There is nothing to fear from turning within and heeding the desires that you hear. Listen for your truth.

Anything Else

People have a lot to say about "living your truth," and it might be fun to take a deep dive into an internet search for this phrase or something similar—or pair it with "yoga" and see what inspiration shows up!

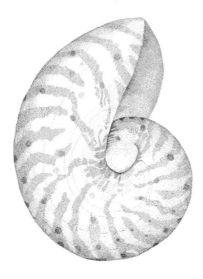

ASTEYA

Write a Little about Your Theme and Why It Speaks to You

Asteya, or "nonstealing," is a pretty basic concept. We are encouraged not to take things that don't belong to us. This plays out on the mat in an interesting way: it can be tempting to overreach and to attempt physical poses that are inappropriate for our bodies in the moment, or in general. This can lead to injury, and thus it directly contradicts the concept of *ahimsa*. It's useful also to think about *asteya* as moving beyond the stealing of just physical objects. You can steal someone's time or energy. You can "steal their thunder." This even happens in a yoga studio space: when one student moves into a challenging pose, other students can feel a shared sense of success, or they can feel envy. While we may not think of that as "stealing" in the most literal sense, it is.

Chants, Quotes, Mantras, Poems, or Songs That Connect

You are enough. You do enough. You have enough.

"Steal My Sunshine" by Len

"Her Hollow Ways" by Danger Mouse and Daniele Luppi

Poses That Work with Your Theme

Explore poses that can be accessed in *kramas* (stages). Move your students slowly from one level to the next, offering a reminder each time to stay with the right version of the pose for them, their levels, and their bodies. Crow Pose can be played with in this way, and so can poses like Sundial or Bird of Paradise.

Distill Your Theme to a Short Sentence or Intention

Don't take things—including poses—that aren't rightfully yours.

Phrases or Sentences to Employ in These Parts of Your Class

OPENING	DURING MOVEMENTS
Asteya (nonstealing) may seem so obvious as to be inapplicable. But there is more that we can steal than just physical objects. Today, look for places you "steal" a pose that may not be the best choice for your body, your energy, your emotional place. Not everything offered in this class is for you. Don't steal poses that do not help you grow.	As we come into this next pose, there are several options. Which one is the one that fully belongs to you? Which one is the one that is given to you—that you don't have to force or take?
DURING PAUSES	**CLOSING**
We rest to replenish our energy. It's in this quiet space that you return to your breath and return to the truth that your practice shows you: you are enough. There is nothing you have to do or take to be enough. There is no pose you have to force yourself into.	When you vibrate with the wholeness that radiates from within, you realize that there's nothing to take because there's nothing you need to be complete. You have arrived in completeness. You are complete now.

Anything Else

This theme may be the most useful in an advanced or power flow class. A mixed-levels class may find that it resonates too.

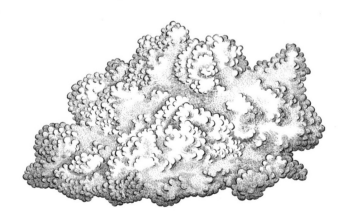

BRAHMACHARYA

Write a Little about Your Theme and Why It Speaks to You

You may have learned in your yoga teacher training that *brahmacharya*, the fourth *yama*, means "sexual chastity." And sure, that's a literal translation. We truly hope this isn't a problem in your yoga classes! To make the concept more applicable, you might use the definition of *brahmacharya* as "temperance," "self-regulation," or "self-control." We like to call it "proper application of energy," because this idea helps guide a physical practice to the appropriate edge, spending energy where it's needed and not where it isn't. It's useful to remind your students that energy, while renewable, is not infinite. We all have a limited supply of energy, and that's especially true for the duration of a yoga practice. *Brahmacharya* is about approaching personal energy with honesty and wisdom.

Chants, Quotes, Mantras, Poems, or Songs That Connect

"It would be a shame to lose the precious jewel of liberation in the mud of ignorant body-building." —K. Pattabhi Jois

"The Journey" by Mary Oliver

"New Soul" by Yael Naïm and David Donatien

Poses That Work with Your Theme

Poses that ask your students to rein it in and do more with less. Great options here are a longer hold in a pose like Bridge Pose, where you take more time to cue subtle ways your student can work harder or choose to relax more. Remind them to practice self-control in their effort.

Distill Your Theme to a Short Sentence or Intention

Is this the right energy for now?

Phrases or Sentences to Employ in These Parts of Your Class

OPENING	DURING MOVEMENTS
Take a moment to scan your body and notice how you're feeling energetically. Are you eager to move? Happy to be still? Are you excited most for the Chaturangas ahead or the blissful Savasana at the end of our class? What do you most need to feel renewed, to feel that your well is full? Move today with a sense of honesty about where you're at and what you need.	How are you using your energy here? Are you being profligate? Could you rein it in?
DURING PAUSES	**CLOSING**
Take this time to reset, breathe, and look again at your well of energy. There is no need to rush through this rest: this is a necessary and important part of our practice too. Allow yourself to luxuriate in this space. The right energy for now is energy of softening and releasing.	The right energy for now is no energy. There is nothing to do. There is no right way to take the space of Savasana. Your practice of *brahmacharya* here is to know that there's nothing to regulate, nothing to control—not even your breath. Let your body be still. Let your mind be still. Do nothing.

Anything Else

There is interesting exploration to be had by acknowledging our modern perspective on this *yama*. Another theme could explore just that: looking at our newer take on *brahmacharya* reminds us that philosophy and political thought isn't timeless. It must evolve to stay relevant and helpful. The same is true of our asana practice. What felt good at twenty may not feel so good at thirty. What felt good on Monday may not feel so good on Friday. Our approach to yoga asana and philosophy must be dynamic, not static, in order to be most helpful.

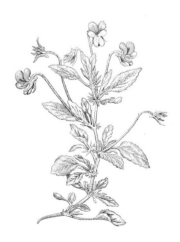

APARIGRAHA

Write a Little about Your Theme and Why It Speaks to You

Aparigraha means "nonhoarding." When we operate from a perspective of scarcity, it can be tempting to protect our resources, because we fear they are finite and not replenishable. If, instead, you consider the gifts you could be sharing with others to be abundant—kindness, positive energy, support, even just a smile—everyone benefits.

Physically, you may be holding back from some postures out of a misguided or fearful sense of self-protection. This can deprive you of potential positive change. When you feel stubborn or immediately come out of a challenging pose, ask yourself whether you are hoarding your energy, and to what end. With appropriate attention to rest, energy is a renewable resource.

Chants, Quotes, Mantras, Poems, or Songs That Connect

"Do your practice and all is coming." —K. Pattabhi Jois

"The places where you have the most resistance are actually the places that are going to be the areas of greatest liberation." —Rodney Yee

"Our True Heritage" by Thich Nhat Hanh

"Try to be a rainbow in someone's cloud." —Maya Angelou

Poses That Work with Your Theme

Standing balance poses, like Warrior III, that put a demand on the muscles but that can be held safely to the very edge of the comfort zone. Chair Pose is great for this too.

Distill Your Theme to a Short Sentence or Intention

Where are you holding back?

Move with abundance.

Phrases or Sentences to Employ in These Parts of Your Class

OPENING

Not all resources are abundant. Money is not. Time is not. But many of the most prized resources in yoga are abundant. Kindness, empathy, and love are renewable, abundant, and even better, they tend to come back to you when you give them away. Let's remember that openness and abundance. Open your eyes and make eye contact with a class member. Smile. Say hi. Let's start our practice from a space of community, remembering that whatever we feel we are lacking, we have kindness, we have love.

DURING MOVEMENTS

When teachers say "shine into the pose," they mean just that: be here fully and abundantly. Be here completely. Don't hold back your energy or your effort. Give all, knowing that there is always more coming. There is nothing to resist. Give all. Shine into the pose.

DURING PAUSES

There is always time to rest and renew, and here we are in that place. When you move in challenging ways, it may feel like there will never be stillness, there will never be relaxation, there will never be a ceasing of the effort. But here we are. Effortless. Know that we always come back to this: rest, space, breath.

CLOSING

With appropriate attention to rest, energy is a renewable resource. Savasana is attention to rest. Take the time to make this an extra restful, extra abundant Savasana by using any props you'd like to add luxury and comfort. Take your rest here as seriously as you took your balancing poses earlier in class. Rest and relaxation are serious business. Give to yourself here, so you can give fully of yourself again later.

Anything Else

If you have a class you trust, adding in a little bit of partner yoga can work nicely for this theme.

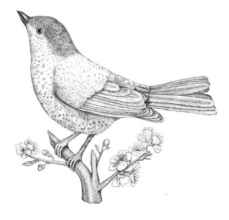

SAUCHA

Write a Little about Your Theme and Why It Speaks to You

Saucha, the first *niyama*, means "cleanliness" or "purity." It's got clear literal application (wash your yoga mat!), but it also applies to asana practice. When we think about cleanliness in movement, we don't necessarily mean strict adherence to alignment. (But if that's the yoga lineage you practice and teach, it certainly *can* mean that too.) Instead, clean movement is movement that is intentional—every aspect of it. Some standard yoga sequences, like Sun Salutations, can get rote. When we're used to moving in routine ways, it can be easy to flow through without full attention to each part of the movement. *Saucha* reminds us that clean yoga is yoga that requires mindfulness. To move cleanly, you have to pay attention.

Chants, Quotes, Mantras, Poems, or Songs That Connect

"Mindfulness isn't difficult, we just need to remember to do it." —Sharon Salzberg

"Constant Surprises" by Little Dragon

"Beginner's Theme Suite" by Brian Reitzell, Roger Neill, and Dave Palmer

Poses That Work with Your Theme

Moving through a sequence your students will know—like Sun Salutations—is a great practice. You can offer them more cues and direction for even the "simple" parts of this sequence. Remind them to spread their fingers and reach as they lift their arms skyward. Remind them to inhale deeply as they lift halfway toward standing. Move through a little slower, offering a reminder to pay attention to all parts. Challenge yourself to offer new cues in familiar poses.

Distill Your Theme to a Short Sentence or Intention

Move with full attention. Practice mindfulness as moving meditation.

Phrases or Sentences to Employ in These Parts of Your Class

OPENING	DURING MOVEMENTS
Let's explore the intention of mindfulness as we move through our practice. Even in yoga—the place where you're trying to learn and cultivate mindfulness—you can end up mindless, flowing through poses with very little attention to how your body feels as you move. Start here, in stillness, cultivating that attention, that clean movement. Breathe cleanly, feeling your belly rise on the inhale, your lungs expand, your body enlivened. As you breathe out, notice your clothes brushing your skin; notice the warmth of your breath on your upper lip; feel the release and softening. Pay attention.	Every breath has your attention. Bring attention into your fingertips. Feel this pose even in your smallest extremities.
DURING PAUSES	CLOSING
Come back to your breath here. Let every breath count. Resting in stillness again, let your attention come fully to how your body feels.	You've just cultivated mindfulness and presence in this practice. Take this clarity, this cleanliness with you as you move off your mat. Stay aware and awake, even as you walk to your car, even as you drive your routine route home.

Anything Else

It can be a fun practice to ask students to move through an established sequence with no cues from you. Perhaps move through it once or twice with them, offering cues and breath reminders. Then ask them to move on their own. Moving in a room with others—but without a teacher leading—can create even more awareness and mindfulness!

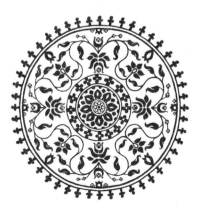

SANTOSHA

Write a Little about Your Theme and Why It Speaks to You

For many of us, looking at the ways we are imperfect and how we can be better or stronger is far more natural than just looking at the ways we are already pretty great. A critical eye serves us well in some environments, but it's exhausting and counterproductive to spend so much time on relentless improvement. *Santosha* reminds us to look at ourselves and find peace and acceptance—a far harder process for some of us. In our yoga practice, *santosha* is about accepting our perceived limitations and, what's more, celebrating them. It's about finding a sense of contentment for where we are in a movement practice, and where we are in an emotional and spiritual practice.

Chants, Quotes, Mantras, Poems, or Songs That Connect

The ocean refuses no river.

So hum ("I am that I am" / "I am divinity")

"Accept everything about yourself—I mean everything. You are you, and that is the beginning and the end—no apologies, no regrets." —Clark Moustakas

"The brain is the hardest part of the body to adjust in asanas." —B. K. S. Iyengar

"The Very First Time" by John Fullbright

Poses That Work with Your Theme

Child's Pose and other resting poses, longer holds in a balance pose (like Dancer Pose), Downward-Facing Dog.

Distill Your Theme to a Short Sentence or Intention

Accept, don't resist.

See the good here.

Phrases or Sentences to Employ in These Parts of Your Class

OPENING	DURING MOVEMENT
Do a body scan. Notice what feels tight, tired, and sore—and notice that is where your attention goes first anyway. But now, notice what already feels good. Notice where your body is already at ease, content, and comfortable.	What would contentment in this pose look like? Can you do less here? The version of the pose you're taking should fulfill your body—no one else's. Look around: see how everyone looks different here? In each pose, we get to compare ourselves to others and see where we're lacking, *or* compare ourselves to others and see the beauty of diversity in the practice of yoga.
DURING REST	**CLOSING**
Find yourself in this moment—breathe—you are here right now. Can you find contentment here? What can you do to feel even more comfortable, content, or at ease here?	Radical contentment is hard work: it involves being vigilant in your response to any voices in your head that tell you that you are not enough as you are. Right now, you are enough. There is nothing to fix here. There is nothing that needs to be done. There is nothing to change or work on. Just be.

Anything Else

It's worth noting that present-day psychological research supports this: the less self-critical we are, the more able we are actually to get stuff done, improve, etc. Self-acceptance is often the first step to change and growth (ironically!).

Self-Compassion by Kristin Neff is a great resource for students who are interested in this theme.

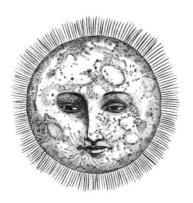

TAPAS

Write a Little about Your Theme and Why It Speaks to You

Tapas is about discipline, zeal, and internal heat. Broadly, we think of it as having the courage to change the things you can—the discipline to take action toward a goal. Without such drive, there's no change, physically, mentally, or spiritually. *Tapas* helps us remember to keep getting on the mat, to keep fighting the good fight. It makes a wonderful theme, as you're preaching to the choir in a group class: they've already taken the step of showing up. Now we parlay that into practice.

Chants, Quotes, Mantras, Poems, or Songs That Connect

"One of Kali's names is 'She who knows the nature of passion.'" —Daniel Odier, *Yoga Spandakarika*

"Kali" by Y La Bamba

"The human being is not a puny speck in this cosmos, as we may appear physically. By virtue of a power called *tapas* ('heat') generated by extreme austerity (also called *tapas*) or in deep stages of meditation, ordinary men or women can compel profound changes in the universe." —Eknath Easwaran, afterword to his translation of The Upanishads

Poses That Work with Your Theme

Any poses that build heat, either through a long hold (think Chair Pose) or through repetition (like a few rounds of Boat!).

Distill Your Theme to a Short Sentence or Intention

Have the courage to change what you can.

Phrases or Sentences to Employ in These Parts of Your Class

OPENING	DURING MOVEMENTS
Here you are: you've taken the biggest step. Set your intention and carry it through your practice with dedication.	Are you shying away from effort? Realign with your intention of discipline.
DURING PAUSES	**CLOSING**
Can you match your effort with release as you rest? Without breaks, you'll be unable to sustain your discipline. Just like day is followed by night, match some ease to your effort.	Rest. Rest with a sense of well-deserved release. Offer gratitude for your effort. What happens on the mat shows us what can happen off the mat. Consider where you might bring the lesson and practice of perseverance into other areas of your life.

Anything Else

Tapas is in a relationship with the two *niyamas: svadhyaya* and *ishvara pranidhana*. Together, they echo the Serenity Prayer: *tapas* is the courage to change what you can, *ishvara pranidhana* is the serenity to accept what you can't change, and *svadhyaya* is the wisdom to know the difference. (Gratitude to Leslie Kaminoff for this lesson.)

A question arises and is especially pertinent on the yoga mat: just because you *can* change something, does that mean that you *should*? Just like fire can be harnessed for good or for bad, *tapas* can be transformative or, unchecked, destructive. Help your students consider what changes are healthy and necessary, and when they may be restless or over-efforting their way into poses, actions, and relationships that don't need changing.

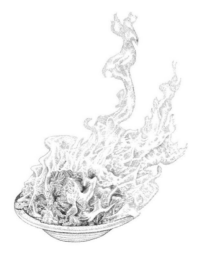

SVADHYAYA

Write a Little about Your Theme and Why It Speaks to You

Self-study is often what brings people to yoga. Yoga offers one path to knowing yourself a bit more, understanding your compulsions and habits, and moving toward a higher, clearer version of yourself. And it's not just something that attracts people to yoga, it's a requisite part of yoga. As one of the *niyamas*, *svadhyaya* tells us that self-study is not optional, it's a requirement. For some of us, this is freeing news. It's exciting to have time and space carved out to get to know yourself more! But for others, it can feel terrifying to turn the magnifying glass inward, as we know full well it will reveal both strengths and weaknesses. Whichever category you land in, gleeful to know yourself more or nervous about digging deeper, there's no way to escape self-study in yoga. Meditating, moving on your mat, and being in community with others all bring growth and reflection.

Chants, Quotes, Mantras, Poems, or Songs That Connect

"Every time you take care of yourself, you're taking care of all of us." —Elena Brower

There's nothing to fear from looking inside. There's nothing to fear from turning within.

"Love after Love" by Derek Walcott

Poses That Work with Your Theme

Child's Pose, a longer Savasana, or restorative poses like Legs Up the Wall or prone bolster twists can offer welcome periods of time for supported meditation.

Distill Your Theme to a Short Sentence or Intention

You're here to learn something about yourself.

Phrases or Sentences to Employ in These Parts of Your Class

OPENING	DURING MOVEMENTS
A lovely side effect of yoga is that you get to know yourself better. You get to know your body as you move. You get to know yourself as you rest in stillness. You get to know your mind as you meditate. We'll spend more time in silence tonight and make even more space for the practice of *svadhyaya*, self-study.	As we come back again to this pose, check in with your mind. What are your assumptions about this pose? What are your assumptions about its ease or challenge? What conversation is your mind having in the background as you move?
DURING PAUSES	CLOSING
In these moments of rest, yoga doesn't stop. It's here that yoga begins. This conversation with yourself is the practice—and it's the most important part of the practice. You're here to learn something about yourself.	As you settle in to rest, soften your face and jaw. Relax the muscles around your eyes. Take a deep, full breath in, and as you exhale, open your mouth and sigh. Move inward. Release.

Anything Else

There is a plethora of smart and funny books out there that can help with *svadhyaya* for interested students. Jen Sincero's *You Are a Badass* is an enjoyable one.

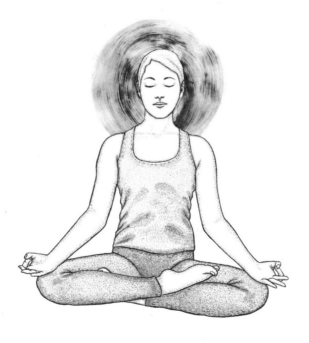

ISHVARA PRANIDHANA

Write a Little about Your Theme and Why It Speaks to You

Ishvara pranidhana means "surrender to the divine." If your students are religious, this will be an easy *niyama* for them to understand. Their connection to the divine may be God. If your students don't follow organized faith, you can talk about broader experiences of the divine. Even atheist yogis can derive a sense of divine by embracing divinity in the wonder of the natural world or in the sacredness of life. Regardless of how *divine* is defined, yoga philosophy encourages us to recognize something larger than ourselves and to surrender to that something. *Yoga* means "union." Surrendering is acknowledging the connection between ourselves and that divine something that is greater than ourselves.

Chants, Quotes, Mantras, Poems, or Songs That Connect

"Spirituality is recognizing and celebrating that we are all inextricably connected to each other by a power greater than all of us, and that our connection to that power and to one another is grounded in love and compassion."
—Brené Brown, *The Gifts of Imperfection*

Let go, let God, or alternatively, Let go, let goodness.

"Canis Lupus" by Alexandre Desplat

Poses That Work with Your Theme

Poses that ask for surrender, like deep hip openers. Poses like Tortoise Pose, splits, and Foot-Behind-the-Head Pose are challenging and humbling. Be sure to teach them with lots of options, especially in a mixed-level class, so your students can surrender without necessarily arriving in the full pose.

Distill Your Theme to a Short Sentence or Intention

You are small by comparison.

Surrender to the divine.

Phrases or Sentences to Employ in These Parts of Your Class

OPENING	DURING MOVEMENTS
Ishvara pranidhana is the tenet of yoga that reminds us that even though our ego *(asmita)* tells us that we are important, we are smaller than the collective. We are smaller than the divine. *Ishvara pranidhana* is a reminder that we alone are not captaining the boat. We might be steering and choosing the route, but we can't control the weather.	Surrender looks like a lot of different things. It looks like surrendering to what your body can do today, right now, without resisting or pushing unsafely.
DURING PAUSES	**CLOSING**
This rest is a momentary surrender. Surrender to the stillness and to your breath. As you breathe with others, remember that you are part of something greater: this community, this world, all of humanity. Notice this divine connection in this small room.	Here, there is nothing to do but to soften and yield. Release, knowing you are safe. You are held. Surrender, knowing there is something more than you.

Anything Else

Luck certainly isn't the same as divinity, but sometimes the concept of luck can remind us that we alone aren't in charge. The article "Why Luck Matters More Than You Think" by Robert H. Frank appeared in *The Atlantic* in May 2016, and it's worth the read.

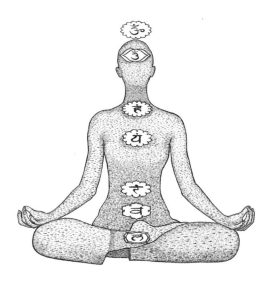

8

THEMING THE SEASONS: SOLSTICES AND EQUINOXES

WINTER SOLSTICE

Write a Little about Your Theme and Why It Speaks to You

The winter solstice represents the shift from darkness into light. As such, it is aligned with a sense of hope, however distant. It's the time of year for nesting and resting, for burrowing into your life and your poses and reconnecting with the quiet and the still. Though the coldest part of winter is ahead, there is more light every day. There will be more every consecutive day.

Chants, Quotes, Mantras, Poems, or Songs That Connect

"New Year Resolve" by May Sarton

"Soon It Will Be Cold Enough" by Emancipator

"Enter One" by Sol Seppy

Poses That Work with Your Theme

Forward folds and other floor poses; restorative poses.

Distill Your Theme to a Short Sentence or Intention

Winter is here; spring is coming.

Let your practice be a light in the darkness.

Phrases or Sentences to Employ in These Parts of Your Class

OPENING	DURING MOVEMENTS
In this week of maximum darkness, how can your practice give you rest and sustenance for the cold months ahead? Can you revel in the darkness and find ease in stillness, while holding faith that more light lies ahead?	Can you find the glimmer of light in this pose, this movement, like a candle in the window on a dark night?
DURING PAUSES	**CLOSING**
Tap into the stillness of the season—even in a time of frantic holiday preparation, the sun is offering us the greatest amount of downtime. Take your rest in this moment.	Can you keep this sense of stillness and presence with you, so that you can confer a little on everyone you come into contact with during the holidays?

Anything Else

The winter season has lots of facets: there's winter in front of the holidays, winter near the New Year, the late winter of graying snow and seemingly never-ending cold. There's a lot to say about all of these faces of winter. Explore this theme, as there may be more to open and unpack here.

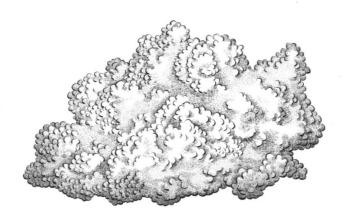

SPRING EQUINOX

Write a Little about Your Theme and Why It Speaks to You

The spring equinox is the time of perfect balance between light and dark. It marks the triumph of light over darkness and is the harbinger of the growth to come. This sense of awakening to the new can bring a fresh perspective to your classes and your own practice. Often, spring weather brings in new students to your classes too. Growth and newness abound. This is the season of hope and renewal.

Chants, Quotes, Mantras, Poems, or Songs That Connect

"We are the change we have been waiting for." —Barack Obama

"The Peace of Wild Things" by Wendell Berry

"Here Comes the Sun" by the Beatles

Poses That Work with Your Theme

Tree Pose! But also anything that moves from grounding to sprouting: Squat to Crow is a good option, or Warrior I to Warrior III, Warrior II to Half Moon, or a lift into Bird of Paradise.

Distill Your Theme to a Short Sentence or Intention

Nurture your intention for growth.

Phrases or Sentences to Employ in These Parts of Your Class

OPENING	DURING MOVEMENTS
As the days' balance shifts from dark to light and the growing season begins, what seeds would you like to plant and see develop over the next few months? Set an intention around nurturing this vision, and let it inform your practice.	Unfurl like a fiddlehead fern opening. Root down, reach up. Lean toward the light.
DURING PAUSES	**CLOSING**
Be sure all your growth is matched with groundedness. The roots are digging into the earth even as the sprouts shoot up.	Commit here to practices that will help you tend the garden of intentions you have set. How can you nurture the seeds you've planted?

Anything Else

The spring equinox has long been celebrated in ancient cultures and faiths. Taking a deeper dive into the traditional themes and celebrations of this season can be a fun way to expand on this theme.

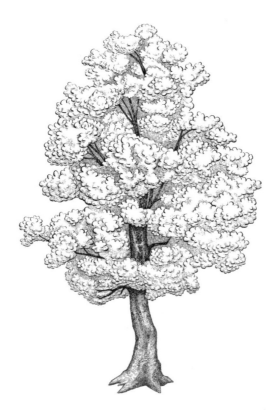

SUMMER SOLSTICE

Write a Little about Your Theme and Why It Speaks to You

The summertime brings with it a feeling of relaxation, joy. Summer is about heat, but it's also about recognition of fullness. Life is at its most alive in the summer!

Chants, Quotes, Mantras, Poems, or Songs That Connect

"Summer afternoon—summer afternoon; to me those have always been the two most beautiful words in the English language." —Henry James

"August 10" by Khruangbin

"Summertime" by George and Ira Gershwin, in any recording you like

Poses That Work with Your Theme

Half Moon Pose, which feels so open and abundant. Five-Pointed Star Pose. Stargazer Pose. You can also lead a light breath-retention practice, guiding students to revel in the fullness between inhalation and exhalation.

Distill Your Theme to a Short Sentence or Intention

Savor the fullness.

Phrases or Sentences to Employ in These Parts of Your Class

OPENING	DURING MOVEMENTS
Let's luxuriate in the abundance of energy and flavor, like we're eating a supper of tomatoes and corn with peaches for dessert.	Find the succulence in this pose, this movement.
DURING PAUSES	**CLOSING**
Summer gives us good reason to rest and relax: the heat makes us want to move slower and savor the moment. So savor this moment. Savor this stillness.	We appreciate summer so much because it feels earned. We've worked through the year. We've made it through the cold of winter. We've arrived halfway through the year, and summer is the time to rejoice in that sense of well-deserved respite. That's Savasana too. You have expended energy in our movement practice, and now your only job is to take a well-deserved rest.

Anything Else

Summer is the time of year when students might have more sporadic attendance, as they travel and get busy with summery things. As you theme summertime classes, keep in mind that your messages have to resonate even more, since your students may not be hearing them as regularly.

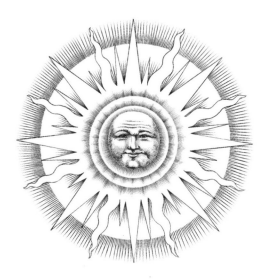

FALL EQUINOX

Write a Little about Your Theme and Why It Speaks to You

Fall is nature's lesson in letting go. Even in the height of the harvest bounty, the signs of change are immanent as the leaves turn colorful and fall and the weather shifts. It's a chance for appreciation of the bounty of the summer, and for preparation for the demands of winter. As such, the fall equinox is a sign to let go of what you don't need, then to stock your metaphorical cellar.

Chants, Quotes, Mantras, Poems, or Songs That Connect

"Wild Geese" by Mary Oliver

"Om" by Hippie Sabotage

"Come Let Go" by Xavier Rudd

Poses That Work with Your Theme

To let go: Breath of Joy. Tree Pose, naturally. Supported poses where the props (including the floor) help you let go of tension.

Distill Your Theme to a Short Sentence or Intention

Let go. Stock up.

Phrases or Sentences to Employ in These Parts of Your Class

OPENING	DURING MOVEMENTS
Even as we delight in the harvest and the fruits of summer, we know we need to store up energy for the winter ahead. In this class, let's practice letting go, turning inward, and stocking up energy.	Are you holding on to excess effort? Consider that trees that don't drop their leaves are more susceptible when the ice storms come early. Let go or be dragged!
DURING PAUSES	**CLOSING**
Settle into the stillness. Bank up your energy in this rest.	See what you've released, as though you are a tree standing tall among a pile of dropped leaves. Turn inward and tap deeply—you already have what you need to get through what comes next.

Anything Else

A beautiful practice to theme in fall might be a restorative practice with expanded focus on letting go.

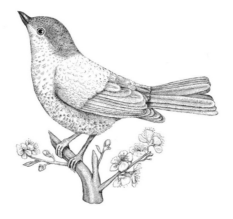

9

OVERCOMING OBSTACLES: BRING THE *KLESHAS* INTO CLASS

AVIDYA

Write a Little about Your Theme and Why It Speaks to You

As the root *klesha,* or cause of suffering, *avidya,* or incorrect seeing, is at the core of all the others. Misperception or wrong vision about how things really are is the base of all struggle. When we learn to see things more clearly, we are witnessing the real, and there is less suffering as a result. Modern visual yoga culture can feed a lot of wrong-seeing and therefore create suffering. We can sometimes see most clearly when we let go of how we think things *should* look and instead intuit our way by how things feel. When you introduce the *kleshas,* students often want to know the solution to each one. For *avidya* (and for all of them, really!) much of the solution is in the yoga practice. Don't we see more clearly after we have moved, breathed, and been in concert with our bodies for an hour? To see more clearly and move to *vidya,* yoga helps.

Chants, Quotes, Mantras, Poems, or Songs That Connect

"Here is my secret. It is very simple: It is only with the heart that one can see rightly; what is essential is invisible to the eye." —Antoine de Saint-Exupéry, *The Little Prince*

"Heart Sutra" by MC Yogi

"The Vacation" by Wendell Berry

Poses That Work with Your Theme

Anything with eyes closed, when it is safe to practice thus.

Distill Your Theme to a Short Sentence or Intention

See clearly; look from your heart.

Phrases or Sentences to Employ in These Parts of Your Class

OPENING	DURING MOVEMENTS
Wrong-seeing or incorrect perception is the heart of suffering. But yoga offers a boon: the asana practice of yoga often clarifies our perception. Moving on your mat creates more open-heartedness. Asana creates essential space that allows you to see things as they truly are.	Take this shape as it is, as you are. Take this shape in the truest way you can, without worries of how it should look.
DURING PAUSES	**CLOSING**
As your breath calms, do you feel a shining from your heart? Do you notice here that already your mind is clearer, your perception sharper?	It is in the rest of Savasana that sometimes the biggest epiphanies of right-seeing appear. As your mind and body rest, notice what subtle messages appear and flicker. Notice what truths get revealed.

Anything Else

Avidya often gets translated as "ignorance," so this is another way to discuss this *klesha*. This ignorance, though, is an ignorance that can be cured. Yoga is the transformative wisdom.

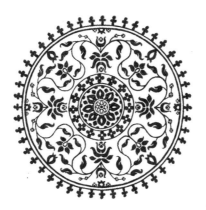

ASMITA

Write a Little about Your Theme and Why It Speaks to You

Asmita refers to the ego, and all its concomitant grandiosity. At heart, overvaluation of the ego is a misperception, and it leads to suffering. You might think of the ego as being a particular pair of glasses through which we are looking at the world. Yoga is a tool to remove those glasses and see reality without ego as the first lens.

Chants, Quotes, Mantras, Poems, or Songs That Connect

> "I understood that the attachment to myself and my image … was actually taking me away from myself, away from this wonderful opportunity to just sit, just breathe, just feel the warm animal of my body." —Stephen Cope, *Yoga and the Quest for the True Self*

> "The Dilemma" by David Budbill

> "Imagine" by John Lennon

Poses That Work with Your Theme

Any poses that allow stillness and space. Legs Up the Wall is a nice option. You could start your class there, as you introduce this theme.

Distill Your Theme to a Short Sentence or Intention

There is more than me.

Phrases or Sentences to Employ in These Parts of Your Class

OPENING	DURING MOVEMENTS
Our practice today gives you the chance to watch how ego shows up everywhere. What happens on your mat reveals what happens off your mat. As we practice, listen for the word "I." When does that show up and get in the way of what is really happening in this room?	What story do you tell yourself about these poses? Do you have a story that begins, "I like this pose" or "I am good at this pose"? Do you have a story that begins "I don't like this pose," or "I can't do this pose"? Look for these fictions to which your ego is so attached. When they arise, notice them. Then do the pose without the story.
DURING PAUSES	CLOSING
Can you be here fully without crafting the experience through the lens of ego? Can you just notice this moment without labeling it or attaching your ego's opinion to it?	Freeing yourself from ego happens in moments. It happens here, as you let go and make room only for release and sensation, not judgment or attachment. Settle into an ego-less rest here, and allow the memory of this to move with you off the mat, so you may find it again.

Anything Else

There is so much written about ego that you could probably craft an entire month of classes around this concept alone.

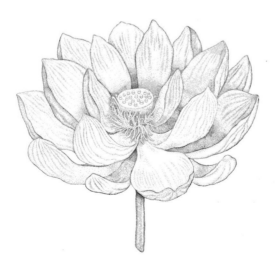

RAGA

Write a Little about Your Theme and Why It Speaks to You

Raga is attachment to the sweet, easy parts of life. On the surface, there's nothing wrong with having preferences for comfort and desires for the things we like. *Raga* becomes a problem when we experience anger, frustration, and sorrow because we can't have what we are attached to. It's the minute annoyance we deal with when, say, our latte isn't made right. But those annoyances can add up and cause a lot of discomfort and suffering if *raga* is allowed to reign unchecked.

Chants, Quotes, Mantras, Poems, or Songs That Connect

Let go.

Moderation in all things.

"My Way" by Calvin Harris

"Om Mani Padme Hum" by Marti Nikko and DJ Drez

Poses That Work with Your Theme

Side Plank, Sundial Pose, any pose that replaces a pose you might usually do, for example, Puppy in place of Child's Pose; Dolphin in place of Downward-Facing Dog. A different transition between poses, such as doing the typical *vinyasa* of Low Push-Up–Upward-Facing Dog–Downward-Facing Dog in reverse. Change it up and thwart attachment.

Distill Your Theme to a Short Sentence or Intention

Question attachment.

Do your attachments cause you joy or suffering?

Phrases or Sentences to Employ in These Parts of Your Class

OPENING	DURING MOVEMENTS
We start our practice in a place of ease. Notice your attachments already here. Are you eager to move or eager to stay? How are these subtle attachments already swaying your experience?	We've changed it up today, and we're doing poses in places we don't normally do them. Has your mind protested? Can you detach from what is expected and preferred and find something valuable in the unusual?
DURING PAUSES	**CLOSING**
Question attachment. Use this time to return to your intention to watch and look for the ways your desires change your experience of reality.	We're taking Savasana in a new way today, as one more way to notice how attachments shift our emotions. You may have already noticed your resistance to this unexpected break from the norm. Can you also notice, though, that even in this different approach, Savasana still brings respite and peace?

Anything Else

Have your students start class or end class in a different way. You could even have them take Savasana with their heads placed on the opposite end of the mat than usual. Anything that causes them to notice their subtle attachments (and challenge them) is good for this theme.

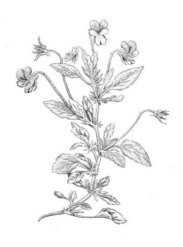

DVESHA

Write a Little about Your Theme and Why It Speaks to You

Dvesha is the opposite of *raga:* while *raga* is attachment to things we like, *dvesha* is aversion to things we don't. We all have things, experiences, and people that we find unpleasant. Like any normal person, you probably try to avoid these things. No one enjoys having to come face to face with unpleasantness. But because life inevitably and regularly makes you confront sources of displeasure, *dvesha* creates suffering. You experience suffering because you are averse to particular (but normal) aspects of life. And as you know from being afraid to watch a horror movie, often *dvesha* magnifies the scary elements into something that's more fearful in imagination than in real life.

Chants, Quotes, Mantras, Poems, or Songs That Connect

"Craving and aversion arise when the senses encounter sense-objects. Do not fall prey to these two brigands blocking your path." —Bhagavad Gita, translation by Stephen Mitchell

"Hallelujah" by Jeff Buckley

"Breathe In Breathe Out" by Mat Kearney

Poses That Work with Your Theme

Try breaking down most-hated poses to make them more accessible. Poll your students at the end of one class to see what poses they would rather avoid, then prep a class or a series of classes to demystify them and make them more accessible and comfortable. Or offer some alternative poses that achieve a similar effect.

Distill Your Theme to a Short Sentence or Intention

Are you causing suffering by fighting what is?

Your mind creates the suffering.

Phrases or Sentences to Employ in These Parts of Your Class

OPENING	DURING MOVEMENTS
Not everything we do today on our mats will be to your liking. If you are a seasoned yoga practitioner, you're probably very clear about the poses you don't like! Today, look for places you are averse to the practice. Look for where you resist and think "I don't like this." Consider how your resistance—not the pose we're doing—causes your suffering.	We're moving into a pose that many of you have expressed not enjoying. Pause here before we try it and challenge yourself to try it with no aversion. Come into the pose from a space that is as neutral as possible. Let that change your experience of the pose.
DURING PAUSES	**CLOSING**
Here, recommit to your intention to move without resistance to any part of the practice.	Do you have aversion to the stillness at the end of class? More reason to stay in Savasana and let the grip of that aversion soften. Often our aversion to something is worse in our imagination than in reality. Be here, allowing what happens to happen.

Anything Else

Buddhism's second noble truth teaches us that attachment causes suffering. The practice of *tonglen* meditation is a lovely way to sensitize yourself to the suffering of others in the service of freeing all from suffering.

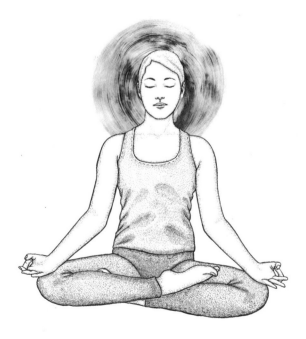

ABHINIVESHA

Write a Little about Your Theme and Why It Speaks to You

The last of the *kleshas* is *abhinivesha,* attachment to life. Death is inevitable, and yoga philosophy, while lofty in moments, keeps us firmly rooted to reality with this tenet. Since death is inevitable and you are going to die, fearing death creates unnecessary suffering. Acceptance that life ends moves us from suffering to freedom. It's helpful to think of the converse to *abhinivesha:* you weren't afraid of what existed before you arrived here, so why have fear of returning to it? With every spike of anxiety about death—your own or the death of your loved ones—*abhinivesha* can serve as a reminder to live fully. If there is no getting out alive, and there is only this one life, well, you'd better embrace the sweetness of the gift while you have it.

Chants, Quotes, Mantras, Poems, or Songs That Connect

"The Self is everywhere. Bright is the Self, Indivisible, untouched by sin, wise, Immanent, and transcendent. He it is Who holds the cosmos together."—Isha Upanishad 8, translated by Eknath Easwaran

"The soul is never born nor does it die." —Bhagavad Gita, translation by Stephen Mitchell

"If We Were Vampires" by Jason Isbell

Poses That Work with Your Theme

Corpse Pose

Distill Your Theme to a Short Sentence or Intention

Death's inevitability is a call to appreciate now.

Phrases or Sentences to Employ in These Parts of Your Class

OPENING	DURING MOVEMENTS
We're looking at a harder yogic truth today: death and our attachment to life. This is not a philosophical challenge that will be resolved with our first approach to it. Rather, conquering *abhinivesha* is a lifelong challenge. But you can start today, now, by seeing this attachment and using it as a reminder to appreciate the sweet life you have now.	Moving and flowing here, you are most alive. As you come into the next pose, find a sense of joy for the simple truth that you are here, alive, breathing, and moving.
DURING PAUSES	**CLOSING**
A yoga practice mimics the cycle of life. We start slowly, build to challenging poses, and then we rest fully. Sometimes along the way, we take a break. That's where we are now: living fully, but pausing to restore.	Everything wants to live. While attachment to life can create anxiety and get in the way of living, recognizing that this attachment exists for all life brings you into harmony with all living creatures. We are all one.

Anything Else

There is much written about this topic, a lot of it serious. On the flip side, David Sedaris had a funny and moving essay in *The New Yorker* in 2006 about remembering that death is inevitable called "Memento Mori."

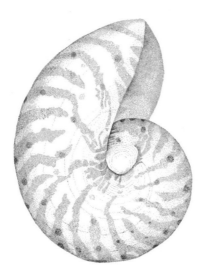

10

YOGA PHILOSOPHY HIGHLIGHTS: ANCIENT THOUGHT AND DAILY LIVING

STHIRA AND *SUKHA*: EFFORT AND EASE

Write a Little about Your Theme and Why It Speaks to You

One of the most central books of yoga thought is The Yoga Sutras by Patanjali, written somewhere around two thousand years ago. In this book—one of the first that compiled yoga philosophy in one place—yoga poses are mentioned only once. Patanjali tells us nothing more than this: yoga poses should be steady and comfortable. That's it.

Stability and freedom are the requirements for a good practice. You must feel strong enough to move in ways that help you, but you must feel fluid and free enough that you aren't building or holding unnecessary tension. This balance between effort and ease is at the heart of every yoga practice—on and off the mat.

Chants, Quotes, Mantras, Poems, or Songs That Connect

"We should endeavor to bring … qualities of gentleness and steadiness to our asana practice, all while making sure that we exert progressively less effort in developing them." —T. K. V. Desikachar, *The Heart of Yoga*

Sthira sukham asanam (Asana is a steady, comfortable posture.) —Yoga Sutra 2.46, translated by Sri Swami Satchidananda

"Gayatri Mantra" by Deva Premal

Poses That Work with Your Theme

Balance poses that require stability and flexibility work so nicely here. Consider Dancer Pose or Revolved Half Moon Pose.

Distill Your Theme to a Short Sentence or Intention

Find the place between effort and ease.

Phrases or Sentences to Employ in These Parts of Your Class

OPENING	DURING MOVEMENTS
The difference between yoga and other forms of movement is that in yoga we move with a clear intention. Our intention today is to find the appropriate balance of effort and ease in this practice.	It's during this part of our practice that you are making the most effort. Making shapes with your body requires focus and energy. But even in the most challenging of poses, look for ways you can soften, do less, and find ease.
DURING PAUSES	**CLOSING**
As we rest, you can find complete ease. Or maybe here there are some spaces in your body that remain "on," engaged, ready to move again. Or maybe your body is at ease, but your mind is stable, strong, and aware. Find the balance.	In Savasana, release any effort to find all ease. Have faith that you are stabilized now by forces outside your body: the floor, gravity, props. Allow your body to fully relax. Find ease.

Anything Else

There are several good translations of The Yoga Sutras. Explore them and find the one that resonates with you. There are many good lessons to take from this text.

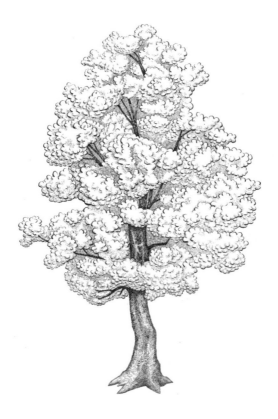

ABHYASA AND *VAIRAGYA*: MAKING AND LETTING

Write a Little about Your Theme and Why It Speaks to You

The Yoga Sutras tell us that we can achieve the state of yoga through a combination of *abhyasa,* or diligent practice, and *vairagya,* or nonattachment to the outcome of this practice. These concepts are simultaneously at odds—effort and dispassion—and intertwined. They echo the injunction, also in the sutras and investigated in the previous theme, that yoga asana should have elements of effort and of ease. In vernacular terminology, we like to think of *abhyasa* and *vairagya* as finding the right balance between making things happen and letting things happen. An asana practice is a laboratory for learning to discern where diligent practice and effort will pay off, and where we must let go of attachment to results. As Kenny Rogers so famously sang, "You've got to know when to hold 'em, know when to fold 'em."

Chants, Quotes, Mantras, Poems, or Songs That Connect

"The General Specific" by Band of Horses

"Comptine d'un autre été: l'après-midi" by Yann Tiersen

Poses That Work with Your Theme

Any standing pose that requires work in the lower body and relaxation in the upper body. Invite students to allow both states at once.

Distill Your Theme to a Short Sentence or Intention

Learn where it's worth making things happen, and where to let things happen.

Phrases or Sentences to Employ in These Parts of Your Class

OPENING	DURING MOVEMENTS
The concept of *abhyasa* encourages us to sustain practice for a long time without interruption. Thank yourself for showing up to continue your practice. At the same time, be aware of any attachment to the outcome of your efforts, and see where you can release this feeling.	What parts of your body need to work here? What parts need to relax? You can often feel this top to bottom in your body, or even front to back: as your back muscles engage in a backbend, for example, the muscles in the front must let go.
DURING PAUSES	**CLOSING**
Honor your effort, release the outcome.	The physical practice is done for now; thank yourself for your efforts. Release completely into rest. As you move into the world, notice where you tend toward a making-things-happen mentality, or where you are passive. Find the right balance between making and letting.

Anything Else

This duality between effort and ease, work and rest plays out across many of our themes, as it is a central concept in yoga and a prime benefit for investigating.

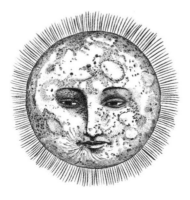

ATHA: AND NOW

Write a Little about Your Theme and Why It Speaks to You

Atha is the first word in the Yoga Sutras. As a rhetorical device, it signals a shift from presentation of the evidence to a summary argument. Given everything that we have already learned and experienced, now begins the study of yoga. It's like a "Hey, y'all: listen up." Think of it as an attention-grabber, like the short announcement that comes on before an HBO show. "And now … the HBO original series, *Ballers*." Hearing that voice say "And now" hustles you from the kitchen onto the couch, serving as a reminder to come and be present in the moment—in the *now*.

Judith Hanson Lasater has said that this is the key word of the Sutras: *now*. Yoga is happening now. Every moment is now. Stay aware; stay connected.

Chants, Quotes, Mantras, Poems, or Songs That Connect

"If you want to conquer the anxiety of life, live in the moment, live in the breath." —Amit Ray

"Both Sides Now" by Joni Mitchell

Poses That Work with Your Theme

Poses that poignantly bring home the idea of now are inversions. They require focus and presence to be in them, but often time slows down when you arrive in them. You can't escape now-ness when you're turned upside down.

Distill Your Theme to a Short Sentence or Intention

Now, now, now.

Phrases or Sentences to Employ in These Parts of Your Class

OPENING	DURING MOVEMENTS
The practice of yoga is a practice of staying present with the now. So often, our minds want to review the past or make guesses about the future. For today's practice, set your intention on now.	When your attention wanders, bring it right back to now. And this now, and this now, and this now.

DURING PAUSES	CLOSING
Feel how the pauses are now too. Feel how your breath is now too.	Take now with you from your mat into the world. There will be times when you're required to think about the future and plan. But always come back to the moment of your breath. Return to the now.

Anything Else

The concept of being in the now is the central tenet of mindfulness. You and your students may already know the book *The Power of Now* by Eckhart Tolle. It's a clear introduction to this concept of being in the present moment.

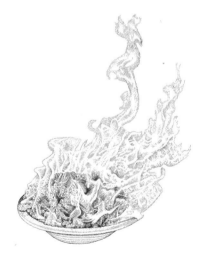

SAMSKARA: GROOVES VERSUS RUTS

Write a Little about Your Theme and Why It Speaks to You

Samskara, or thought impressions, are the patterns we adopt and repeat over a lifetime. The concept of *samskara* explains that every action leaves a record in the psyche, like footsteps in a snowy field. These records can be positive or negative. Think of the positive *samskara* as a groove: a good habit that, repeated regularly, leads to good outcomes. For example, engaging in healthy behavior like eating well and exercising is a good groove to be in. But other habits are not useful grooves but instead ruts—they are cut deeply and followed without a chance of deviation, and they can be harmful. While healthy behavior can have a life-enhancing benefit, it can also change from a groove to a rut and become the harmful condition of orthorexia. Or a movement we take in an *asana* practice—say, Chaturanga—can be helpful in small doses but harmful when practiced too much over time. Our practice can form either a groove or a rut; self-study and continual attention to whether our habits are currently helpful are key.

Chants, Quotes, Mantras, Poems, or Songs That Connect

"I Am Already" by Danna Faulds

"Groove Me" by King Floyd

"Groove Is in the Heart" by Deee-Lite

Poses That Work with Your Theme

Any new approach—whether in your cueing, in the pose from which you approach a familiar pose, or in a new orientation in the room—will help students notice their habits, which is the first step to changing them.

Distill Your Theme to a Short Sentence or Intention

Is this pattern a groove or a rut?

Phrases or Sentences to Employ in These Parts of Your Class

OPENING	DURING MOVEMENTS
Notice the habits manifest in your body as you sit for centering. Is one leg always on top or in front? Does your posture carry the record of your office chair and car seat?	Pay attention to the feelings here. Are you traveling the path of least resistance, so that your movement is free and easy? Or do you find yourself in a rut, moving mindlessly or traveling on a bumpy path?
DURING PAUSES	CLOSING
Notice the habitual patterns of your mind—the *chitta vritti*. Are they useful to you now?	Every moment is a chance to create a new *samskara* that serves you now.

Anything Else

Students who like this idea of finding a groove and breaking a rut might find more wisdom in the book *Unfu*k Yourself* by Gary John Bishop.

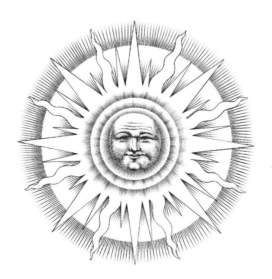

ACTION WITHOUT ATTACHMENT TO RESULTS

Write a Little about Your Theme and Why It Speaks to You

In The Bhagavad Gita, Krishna tells Arjuna, "You have right to your actions but never to your actions' fruits. Act for the action's sake. And do not be attached to inaction. Self-possessed, resolute, act without any thought of results, open to success or failure. This equanimity is yoga" (translation by Stephen Mitchell). This message is counter to much of what modern culture tells us about self-worth: it's only achievable with measurable success. But Krishna speaks an important truth in the Gita. Our worth isn't measured in the outcome; it's measured in our effort.

Chants, Quotes, Mantras, Poems, or Songs That Connect

Act without any thought of results.

Prelude in G Minor, Opus 23, No. 5, by Sergei Rachmaninoff

"Namah Shivaya" by Krishna Das

Poses That Work with Your Theme

A challenging pose like full split or Visvamitrasana is a good one to explore. There are lots of opportunities for doing similar poses that lead to these peak poses, which works well with this theme.

Distill Your Theme to a Short Sentence or Intention

Do your duty with no attachment to results.

Phrases or Sentences to Employ in These Parts of Your Class

OPENING	DURING MOVEMENTS
You've come to yoga today, and your duty for this practice is to be in your body, with your breath, making shapes. There's nothing you have to achieve with those shapes—no final form you have to take. The important part of our practice is to make an effort without necessarily attaining anything. Off the mat, many of us struggle with this. How often do we want to work hard without a guarantee that it will get us something?	Do what you can here. There's nothing that has to happen. Make your best effort, knowing that the effort is the goal.
DURING PAUSES	**CLOSING**
Rest takes effort too. For many of us, with abundant energy and anxiety, resting fully takes the most effort. Even if there isn't a full letting go here, make the attempt.	Doing your duty without attachment to results by necessity means that you first have to define your duty. Sometimes that's easy, in the context of being a parent or in a job environment. But often, your duty in life is a more amorphous, undefined thing. It's asking yourself, "What am I here for?" and "What am I supposed to give?" When you find the answers, do your duty.

Anything Else

Again, we see the tenets of Buddhism running parallel to yoga philosophy. The third noble truth teaches that nonattachment leads to freedom from suffering.

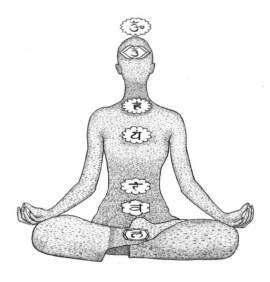

THE *GUNAS*

Write a Little about Your Theme and Why It Speaks to You

In Ayurvedic thinking, all *prakriti* (matter) in the universe is made up of *gunas* or qualities in varying amounts. These qualities are *tamas, rajas,* and *sattva. Tamas* is the state of darkness and stagnation. *Rajas* is the state of action and movement. *Sattva* is the state of harmony and balance. It is the practice of yoga that brings a more sattvic life. It's hard to hold in our black-or-white minds that something can have qualities of all three: inertia, energy, and balance. But indeed, isn't a lovely yoga practice exactly that? There is space for rest, space to move, and those two together help us achieve a greater sense of equilibrium.

Chants, Quotes, Mantras, Poems, or Songs That Connect

"In the attitude of silence, the soul finds the path in a clearer light, and what is elusive and deceptive resolves itself into crystal clearness."
—Mahatma Gandhi

"Darkness cannot drive out darkness; only light can do that. Hate cannot drive out hate; only love can do that." —Martin Luther King Jr.

"Everything's Not Lost" by Coldplay

Poses That Work with Your Theme

For this theme, build a sequence that moves with intention from stillness to flow back to stillness to cultivate harmony.

Distill Your Theme to a Short Sentence or Intention

Move toward *sattva,* the state of harmony.

Phrases or Sentences to Employ in These Parts of Your Class

OPENING All matter is made up of parts that are stagnant, parts that are dynamic, parts that are stable—all matter including you. While all of this exists at once inside you, you can shape this matter toward stability and harmony. We'll move with that intention today.	**DURING MOVEMENTS** Don't force the poses. And don't be indolent in the poses. Let your movements have a harmony to them.
DURING PAUSES This is rest, but it's not stagnation. It's preparation for what's coming next. It's the necessary downtime for the energy you expend. This pause creates symmetry in the practice.	**CLOSING** Leave your mat knowing that you are all things—dark, moving, balanced—and that through your practice today, you moved your energy into greater harmony.

Anything Else

It can be tempting to favor one *guna* over the others—to think that *tamas* is negative, for example. Fight this urge: all of the elements are important for balance.

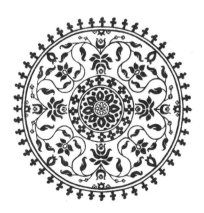

THE *VAYUS*

Write a Little about Your Theme and Why It Speaks to You

The word *vayu* means "wind," but that doesn't fully confer the idea behind the *vayus*. *Prana*, or energetic life force, can move and function in different ways: the five *vayus* are those ways. Instead of cuing students to press their feet downward, teachers can suggest that students look for and harness the movement of *apana vayu*, for instance downward-flowing *prana*. The five *vayus* are *prana vayu*, which flows in and up and is associated with the consumption of food, water, and breath; *apana vayu*, which flows downward and is associated with elimination, menstruation, and childbirth; *samana vayu*, which flows toward the body center and is associated with digestion; *vyana vayu*, which flows away from the body center and is associated with the spread of breath and life force through the body; and *udana vayu*, which flows up and outward and is associated with singing, chanting, exhalation, and speech. Teaching about the *vayus* and encouraging students to look at the way energy moves in their own bodies is especially important in helping them to tune into the subtleties of the practice.

Chants, Quotes, Mantras, Poems, or Songs That Connect

"All forms of *prana* are necessary, but to be effective, they must be in a state of balance with each other." —T. K. V. Desikachar, *The Heart of Yoga*

"Breath is a bridge which connects life to consciousness, which unites your body to your thoughts." —Thich Nhat Hanh, *The Miracle of Mindfulness*

"Breath Control" by MC Yogi

Poses That Work with Your Theme

Any poses work, but think in advance about how you might cue poses in connection to the *vayus*. Here are some that fit nicely: chanting "om" for *udana vayu*; radiating out in a pose like Warrior II for *vyana vayu*; engaging core in an arm balance for *samana vayu*; noticing breath for *prana vayu* (or specific *pranayama* practices); and directing energy downward in a pose like Squat for *apana vayu*.

Distill Your Theme to a Short Sentence or Intention

You are more than a body; you are a container for *prana*, life force.

Feel the way that energy moves in you.

Phrases or Sentences to Employ in These Parts of Your Class

OPENING	DURING MOVEMENTS
We start in stillness, but even here, *prana* is moving. It's moving in deep ways in your body, stimulating digestion and flooding your cells with breath. Watch your breath. *Prana vayu* is here: breath flows in, filling your lungs. *Vyana vayu* brings this fresh energy to all your limbs, your smallest fingers and toes. As you breathe in stillness, feel this radiating energy.	As you arrive in [a pose], lift your heart skyward and feel the energy of your body radiate from your chest outward. Extend your arms away from your body, feeling this action as physical, but also as energetic: *prana* flowing from your heart center toward your fingertips.
DURING PAUSES	**CLOSING**
As you come back to your breath in this in-between space, come back also to the flow of *prana*. Breath in, breath out. Life in each breath.	Your corporeal body moves as you move, and your subtle body pulses and swirls in movement and stillness. Energy is always active in you, even here, back in calm tranquility. As you rest in stillness, become aware of this energy in you, in the room, in the others near you. Let your body breathe, knowing breath is so much more than air: it's life.

Anything Else

You might find, as we have, that students are really interested in this idea, but that one class is not quite enough exposure for them to fully grasp it. Consider theming the *vayus* for a month of classes, and drawing your students' attention to a specific *vayu* in each class.

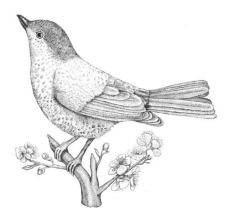

THE *DOSHAS: VATA*

Write a Little about Your Theme and Why It Speaks to You

The three *doshas* described in Ayurveda—*vata, pitta,* and *kapha*—are present in all of us. Most of us tend to skew toward one or the other. We are *vata,* which means we are creative and full of air element; or we are *pitta,* fiery and full of fire element; or we are *kapha,* grounded with the earth element. Each of these *doshas* is important for balance, and having harmony among them while recognizing which way we naturally skew will promote optimal health. The lens of the *doshas* is a tool for self-awareness.

Theming *vata dosha* means connecting to all that is airy, creative, energetic, and spontaneous. *Doshas* can be in harmony or out of balance. When *vata dosha* is out of balance, the result is discombobulation, confusion, and anxiety. But *vata* in harmony delights in creative expression and discovery. Discuss this *dosha,* reminding students to connect to the creative and spontaneous in themselves.

Chants, Quotes, Mantras, Poems, or Songs That Connect

"We have to continually be jumping off cliffs and developing our wings on the way down." —Kurt Vonnegut, *If This Isn't Nice, What Is?*

"Voilà" by Jeanne Cherhal

"Silver Clouds" by the Bowerbirds

Poses That Work with Your Theme

A practice themed around *vata dosha* can be fluid, changing, and have varied expressions of poses. In longer holds of poses, offer students options so they have more choice. You might also set aside a section of class that is uncued, so students can have free rein to do their own practice. With its creative alignment, Wild Thing is a fun pose to include.

Distill Your Theme to a Short Sentence or Intention

Let your spirit flow unchecked.

Phrases or Sentences to Employ in These Parts of Your Class

OPENING	DURING MOVEMENTS
All of us have all elements in us. In our practice tonight, we'll move with creativity and fluidity, moving away from precision and trusting intuition to guide us as we move. Let's move with curiosity, delight, and free spiritedness.	Choose a playful variation on this form. You might sway your arm, lift your heart, or sweep your leg out. If you can, close your eyes or lower your gaze and explore adding creative movement without looking. Connect to the creative force inside.
DURING PAUSES	**CLOSING**
Even here, find a unique expression of this pose.	Revel in the joyous shapes that your free-flowing form created! Relax now, knowing that your creativity is stoked, and your lightness as a being has been reignited. As you move back into the world from this practice, bring the airiness and freedom of *vata* with you.

Anything Else

We like the book *Yoga and Ayurveda* by David Frawley for a fuller exploration of *dosha* types and how the ancient medicine of Ayurveda and yoga intersect. In addition, students who are interested in *dosha* types and are curious about their own will find an abundance of *dosha* constitution quizzes online.

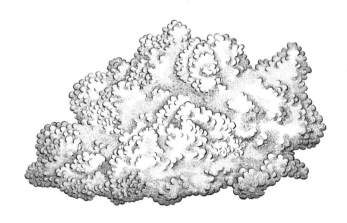

THE *DOSHAS: PITTA*

Write a Little about Your Theme and Why It Speaks to You

Pitta, fiery and full of fire element, is the *dosha* type associated with leadership, decisiveness, directness, and resilience. Out of harmony, *pitta dosha* can be jealous or angry, a fire that rages without relief. But in balance, *pitta* constitution confers strength, precision, intellect, and concentration. It's helpful to remind students that in our very chaotic and changing world, they can remain unswayed, true to themselves, and focused.

Chants, Quotes, Mantras, Poems, or Songs That Connect

"The wise man lets go of all results, whether good or bad, and is focused on the action alone. Yoga is skill in action." —Bhagavad Gita, translation by Stephen Mitchell

"Burn It in the Fire" by Wade Morissette

Poses That Work with Your Theme

A *pitta dosha* practice should include heat-generating movements and active *vinyasa*. Poses that require fire and concentration are good options. Elbow Plank, Forearm Balance, and Crow Pose would fit nicely.

Distill Your Theme to a Short Sentence or Intention

Find your fire.

Phrases or Sentences to Employ in These Parts of Your Class

OPENING	DURING MOVEMENTS
We'll move from a *pitta* place today. Bring concision into your alignment. Bring determination into your form. Move today with grit and focus, stoking your inner fire.	Notice the physical challenge of this pose, and meet it with your mental and spiritual determination to be here, fully, present, and to give your full effort.
DURING PAUSES	**CLOSING**
Having internal fire and focus doesn't mean going without rest. To have the energy and determination you want, you must resolve to have self-care, space for renewal, and respite too.	Arrive here most fully, most present. Let every part of your body vibrate with energy and aliveness as you rest, renewed in your capacities.

Anything Else

Balance a fiery practice with a longer rest or something luxurious, like essential oil anointment in Savasana.

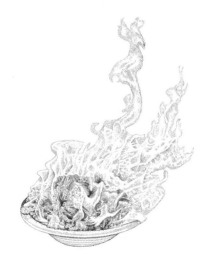

THE *DOSHAS: KAPHA*

Write a Little about Your Theme and Why It Speaks to You

Kapha dosha is grounded with the earth element. *Kapha dosha* is associated with stability, staying power, and home. It's the *dosha* of rest and calm, the *dosha* of patience, support, and loyalty. Out of balance, *kapha dosha* can be static and stubborn. But in balance, this *dosha* is the one that creates the most grounding and safety.

Chants, Quotes, Mantras, Poems, or Songs That Connect

"Goin' Home" by Dan Auerbach

"You Can Always Come to Me" by Greg Brown

Poses That Work with Your Theme

Long holds of poses that challenge the lower body, as well as mellow floor work. Goddess Pose and any variation on squatting work nicely.

Distill Your Theme to a Short Sentence or Intention

Root down.

Get grounded.

Phrases or Sentences to Employ in These Parts of Your Class

OPENING	DURING MOVEMENTS
Focus on your breath here, as a way to connect to your deepest self, in this moment. Feel your body settled here, relaxed here, grounded from this first moment of the practice. Move from this place of rootedness.	Move slow, with attention to the placement of each part of your body. Feel heavy in the pose. Notice the connection of your feet to the ground. As you push the ground away, notice that it rises up to meet you, support you.
DURING PAUSES	**CLOSING**
We'll rest here longer than usual, reconnecting to our breath, and allowing our bodies to relax more fully before we move again. This rest pose is our home base pose, and we will return to it again in this practice.	Grow heavy, and heavier still. Rest with the confidence of complete support from the floor and your props. [It would be a lovely practice here to walk students through relaxing each part of their body, from toes to skull.]

Anything Else

Just as you might have a negative reaction to *tamas,* one of the *gunas,* you may be tempted to revile the *kapha* elements in yourself. Don't! Each of the *doshas* is important and useful. Moving, both literally on the mat and metaphorically through life, from a place of groundedness is paramount to success in all endeavors. You must have a full sense of where you are starting from to arrive at where you want to be.

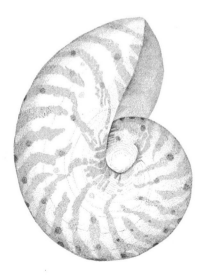

THE *KOSHAS*

Write a Little about Your Theme and Why It Speaks to You

We like to envision the *koshas*, or energetic sheaths of the body, as lampshades that surround the central light within. From the outside in, the *koshas* are the physical body *(annamaya kosha)*, the breath body or energetic body *(pranamaya kosha)*, the thinking body *(manomaya kosha)*, the emotional or wisdom body *(vijnanamaya kosha)*, and the bliss body *(anandamaya kosha)*. When there is harmony among these layers, we shine, like a lamp with intricately cut-out shades all in alignment; it's also typical to be stuck with a hang-up in one or more of them and cast a lower light.

Chants, Quotes, Mantras, Poems, or Songs That Connect

"You do not become good by trying to be good, but by finding the goodness that is already within you and allowing that goodness to emerge." —Eckhart Tolle

"This Little Light of Mine" by Sam Cooke

"At the end of the day, it doesn't matter if you have three out of four of your limbs; it doesn't matter if you're fat, short, tall, male, female, or somewhere in between. None of that matters. All that matters is that we're human and trying to breathe together." —Jessamyn Stanley

Poses That Work with Your Theme

Anything at all! Draw your students' attention to the full experience in each pose: not only in the physical body, but in the breath, in the thoughts, in the feelings, and in the light at center.

Distill Your Theme to a Short Sentence or Intention

Align and shine.

Phrases or Sentences to Employ in These Parts of Your Class

OPENING	DURING MOVEMENTS
We know that yoga goes beyond the poses. Inherent in each shape that the physical body takes is an experience in the breath, in the mind, and in the heart. When these are aligned well—when you are aware of and present to the experience on every level—each pose is a soul-shining experience. Let's see if we can put this into play today. Start by tuning in to every layer, or *kosha*.	Notice where your awareness is. Are you focused only on the external, the physical? Can you connect with breath? And can you also be aware of the experience in your head and your heart as you move? Let your bliss light shine through.
DURING PAUSES	CLOSING
Check back in with the layers of your being. How does taking this rest give them the space to align?	As you move off the mat, carry this self-awareness and alignment into the world.

Anything Else

Yoga nidra, a form of guided meditation, systematically works through the layers of the *koshas.* For more on this lovely practice, see Richard Miller's work and the book *Yoga Nidra* by Swami Satyananda Saraswati.

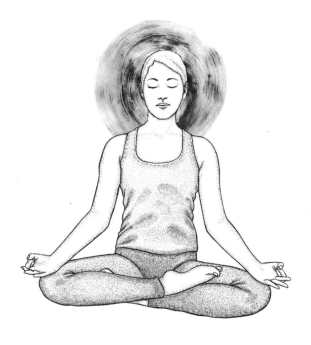

THE CHAKRAS

Write a Little about Your Theme and Why It Speaks to You

Each chakra can be the germ of a theme on its own—perhaps that's where you'd like to start your journaling in part 3. Taken together, the chakras create an inner roadmap for awareness in the body. When all chakras are aligned and tuned, energy flows freely. The chakras are a helpful way to think about modern-day spiritual ailments, metaphorical though they may be.

Chants, Quotes, Mantras, Poems, or Songs That Connect

"Strength, love, courage, love, kindness, love, that is really what matters. There has always been evil, and there will always be evil. But there has always been good, and there is good now." —Dr. Maya Angelou

Chakra mantra (Lam, Vam, Ram, Yam, Ham, Om, resonate sound, silence)

Poses That Work with Your Theme

Consider connecting each chakra to a corresponding pose. Garland Squat or Easy Seated Pose can connect to the root chakra, a heart-opening pose like Camel can connect to the heart chakra, and Headstand can connect to the crown chakra, for instance.

Distill Your Theme to a Short Sentence or Intention

Let energy flow freely.

Phrases or Sentences to Employ in These Parts of Your Class

OPENING	DURING MOVEMENTS
In Ayurveda, there are seven energetic centers in our bodies, the chakras. In our practice today, we'll meditate on each one, connecting a pose to each chakra space and moving with the intention to allow energy to freely flow.	Imagine that energy is flowing from your root to your head. Breathe deeply, allowing nothing to be stuck, nothing to be forced.
DURING PAUSES	**CLOSING**
In places of rest, we gain energy again. Rest, and tune in to the flow of your personal energy when your body is still.	An awareness of your chakras can start you on a path of self-discovery. Allow this knowledge to ignite your interest in self-study and personal growth. The chakras are one more path to deeper self-knowledge.

Anything Else

A class that themes on the chakras as a whole (rather than on one individually) may serve as an introduction to the concept for your students. Don't feel that you have to go to deeply all at once. You might teach a class on the concept of the chakras, and in subsequent classes you could further explore each chakra.

The book *Eastern Body, Western Mind* by Anodea Judith is a nice resource for discussing the chakras and how they fit with our modern-day understanding of psychology.

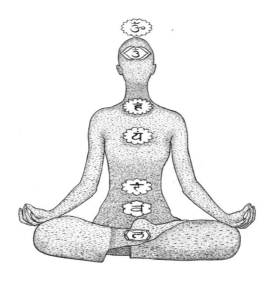

11

WHEN SOMEONE ELSE SAYS IT BEST: QUOTES AS THEMES

.... **"BETWEEN STIMULUS AND RESPONSE THERE IS A** ....
SPACE. IN THAT SPACE IS OUR POWER TO CHOOSE
OUR RESPONSE. IN OUR RESPONSE LIES OUR
GROWTH AND OUR FREEDOM."

—VICTOR FRANKL

Write a Little about Your Theme and Why It Speaks to You

Much of what we're doing in yoga and meditation is about widening the space between stimulus and response so that our experience of being a human in the world is one that is less akin to being a plastic bag blown about by the wind and more similar to being a tree that can weather the changing seasons—shifted, changed, but steady. Frankl's quote taps into that idea and reminds us that the space already exists for all of us. Yoga gives us the capacity to be present to this space, and to understand it is our way to a blissful life.

Chants, Quotes, Mantras, Poems, or Songs That Connect

"Freedom! '90" by George Michael

"Clair de Lune" by Claude Debussy

"Mother of Us All" by Stephen Levine

Poses That Work with Your Theme

Seated meditation at the end of class, so that you may discuss this theme and then allow your students to experience it.

Distill Your Theme to a Short Sentence or Intention

Look for the space between what happens in the world and how you respond.

Look for the space.

Phrases or Sentences to Employ in These Parts of Your Class

OPENING	DURING MOVEMENTS
Settle into your body and start to tune into the space inside that you know is there, but you don't always get a chance to access in our busy world. Breathe deeply and say hello to this interior you—the you that remains unchanged by all that happens in the world. As we move, return to this.	Why does movement in a yoga class give us greater ability to choose our response to the world? In every movement, pose, and breath, you are getting to know yourself more, you are creating more of a connection to yourself. You are deepening your ability to access the secret, quiet space inside.
DURING PAUSES	**CLOSING**
Come back to your deepest self here. Connect to the interior as you breathe.	As you leave this space, vow to nurture this connection to your deeper self. Return to it through your day, your week, knowing that when you come back to the deepest part of yourself, you're cultivating a clearer path to happiness.

Anything Else

Victor Frankl's *Man's Search for Meaning* is a book worth reading—and it will certainly inspire more themes.

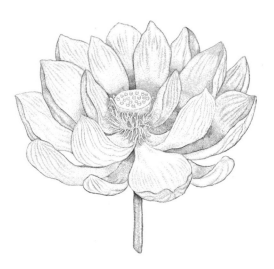

·················   **"THE APPEARANCE OF THINGS CHANGES**   ·················
ACCORDING TO THE EMOTIONS; AND THUS WE SEE
MAGIC AND BEAUTY IN THEM, WHILE THE MAGIC
AND BEAUTY ARE REALLY IN OURSELVES."

—KAHLIL GIBRAN

Write a Little about Your Theme and Why It Speaks to You

Gibran's quote reminds us that again, the external world and the internal experience are not always aligned. Whether we see a magical and beautiful world has more to do with the emotional lens we're looking through than anything else. We can create our own meaning, magic, and beauty, but we have to believe that it's in our power to do so.

Chants, Quotes, Mantras, Poems, or Songs That Connect

"Follow the Sun" by Xavier Rudd

"Cherokee Morning Song" by Robbie Robertson

Yogas chitta vritti nirodha (Yoga is the quieting of the mind's fluctuations.)
—Yoga Sutra 1.2

Poses That Work with Your Theme

Cue poses that you don't usually cue. Stay away from the more routine poses you teach, and try something that may feel new and magical and give students a fresh perspective on their practice.

Distill Your Theme to a Short Sentence or Intention

You create your own magic.

Phrases or Sentences to Employ in These Parts of Your Class

OPENING	DURING MOVEMENTS
Our emotions change our experience of the world. When we're happy, the world seems brighter—we notice the good. When we're troubled, the world echoes that sentiment, and we notice all the darkness. Acknowledge to yourself now how you feel today. How have you arrived on your mat? What is your mood, energy? What are your expectations? How does this—where you are emotionally—shape your practice?	Whatever experience you're having in this pose is valid. But your experience is shaped by so many things apart from what is happening immediately. Your experience of this pose is shaped by your childhood, what you had for breakfast, the conversation you had right before class. Knowing this, accept your experience of this pose today. It will change tomorrow.
DURING PAUSES	**CLOSING**
Your mind creates your experience—pleasurable or painful. Your mind is the veil between reality and the way you see reality.	Move off your mat with more patience for the fluctuations of your emotions and more patience with your changing feelings toward the world. Your emotions shift, and your view shifts with them. But the magic and beauty of the world is always there, waiting to be seen.

Anything Else

Have you heard that what irritates you about others is probably something you dislike in yourself? This quote flips the same concept into a positive realm.

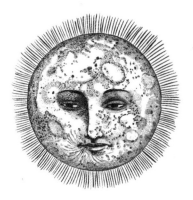

"ARGUE FOR YOUR LIMITATIONS, AND SURE ENOUGH, THEY'RE YOURS."

—RICHARD BACH

Write a Little about Your Theme and Why It Speaks to You

So often things are true simply because we believe they are. "I can't lift to wheel pose," you tell yourself, and of course you can't. And while some limitations are real—sometimes imposed by anatomy in yoga asana, for instance—many are not. This theme is a reminder that we can only do what we believe we can do.

Chants, Quotes, Mantras, Poems, or Songs That Connect

"Faith" performed by Stevie Wonder

"Volunteers" by Megafaun

"Everything has boundaries. The same holds true with thought. You shouldn't fear boundaries, but you should not be afraid of destroying them. That's what is most important if you want to be free: respect for and exasperation with boundaries." —Haruki Murakami, *Colorless Tsukuru Tazaki and His Years of Pilgrimage*

Poses That Work with Your Theme

Any pose that takes a certain amount of courage for your class. Depending on your class and their level, this could be an arm balance like Crow, an inversion, or even something like Warrior III. Choose what will be a manageable challenge for your class and be sure to stress that willingness to attempt the pose (not necessarily complete it) is the success.

Distill Your Theme to a Short Sentence or Intention

Are your limitations self-imposed?

Phrases or Sentences to Employ in These Parts of Your Class

OPENING	DURING MOVEMENTS
We're going to try a pose today that may seem scary, new, or out of your comfort zone. That's the point! We'll build to this pose slowly, and we'll move into it safely and with lots of modifications. We're moving today with belief, though. As you breathe and flow, do so with reverence for your capabilities. There is nothing you have to do, and there is nothing you get if you come fully into the pose. But by trying the pose, at least, you awaken to the fact that you are a vibrant being capable of anything you set out to do. The success is in the trying.	Let's move into our pose now. You have the tools to explore safely. There is so much to learn just by trying. What holds you back here? Fear of injury? Can you do [modified version or alternative pose] instead and find success there? Or try setting up in our pose and just exploring the setup, without even attempting. [Try talking your students into challenging poses using a different set of cues than your regular ones. Or try not mentioning the names of poses at all; just talk them in through cues.]
DURING PAUSES	**CLOSING**
Let's take a rest here, after our attempt at [pose]. Here you are: still you, but with a new awakening to what you're willing to try. You can stretch farther and find more, opening past boundaries that you don't need. In rest, we find the balance to our challenge.	Sit with your success. Sit with your abilities. Sit with your heart more fully open to all that you can do.

Anything Else

Definitely stress to students that self-care and concern about injury are legitimate reasons to opt out of any particular asana offered. That makes teaching this theme a rather sophisticated endeavor: you must both encourage students to challenge perceived limitations and respect real ones.

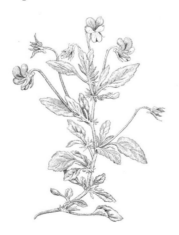

"LOVE IS THE EXTREMELY DIFFICULT REALIZATION THAT SOMETHING OTHER THAN ONESELF IS REAL."

—IRIS MURDOCH

Write a Little about Your Theme and Why It Speaks to You

This beautiful quote speaks to the truth of loving another person: real love transcends ego. And ego is awfully hard to transcend. To love someone fully is to acknowledge the realness of their emotions and to feel compassion toward their experience. While we might imagine that our love for our dearest ones is unceasing, moments of this true experience of love are more fleeting. When we truly see someone, we love them fully. But how often are we able to truly see?

Chants, Quotes, Mantras, Poems, or Songs That Connect

"Love seems to be something that keeps filling up within us. The more we give away, the more we have to give." —Fred Rogers

"Sea of Love" by Cat Power

"Equality is understanding that there is nothing and no one in the universe more important than you. And there is nothing and no one in the universe less important than you." —Gary Zukav

Poses That Work with Your Theme

Heart-opening poses of surrender. Child's Pose.

Distill Your Theme to a Short Sentence or Intention

Real love requires full seeing.

Phrases or Sentences to Employ in These Parts of Your Class

OPENING	DURING MOVEMENTS
This quote acknowledges to us the challenge of real love. Love requires a full arrival in someone else's presence. It requires an acknowledgment that another person also experiences the richness and vastness that you experience personally.	Move with love, with an open heart. Move with a determination to see fully.
DURING PAUSES	**CLOSING**
At the heart of love, then, is compassion. Begin here, in rest, with compassion for yourself. Take the time you need here to care for your body and reset. Extend compassion to yourself, so that you may extend compassion to others.	As you move into rest, imagine your most sacred loved one in your mind's eye. Sit with the experience of your loved one fully, radiating love and gratitude to them.

Anything Else

It would be a fitting practice to pair this theme with *metta* (loving kindness) meditation.

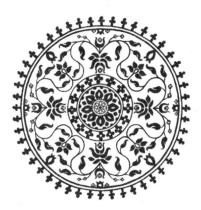

"ABOVE ALL, BE THE HEROINE OF YOUR LIFE, NOT THE VICTIM."

—NORA EPHRON

Write a Little about Your Theme and Why It Speaks to You

Ephron's quote gives us a chance to see that victimhood is sometimes a choice—a way we're choosing to frame our personal narrative. Victimization *is* real and often occurs because of circumstances beyond our control. Not all oppression is equal, and we're not suggesting anyone should make light of systematic cultural oppression. Yet, being victimized *is* a great equalizer: it isn't a unique circumstance. Everyone is a victim at some point. It's not a pleasant, comfortable, or safe role. But it also doesn't have to be a defining one. "Above all, be the heroine of your life, not the victim," because despite circumstances, despite limited power over much of your life, despite your family, wealth, health, or background, *the perspective you choose* plays an important role in your narrative. Your perspective, your personal choice, can help determine if you're going to be the victim or hero of your life story.

Chants, Quotes, Mantras, Poems, or Songs That Connect

"To win a battle, a general surveys the terrain and the enemy and plans countermeasures. In a similar way, the Yogi plans the conquest of the Self."
—B. K. S. Iyengar, *Light on Yoga*

"Strength, Courage, and Wisdom" by India.Arie

No victims, just volunteers.

Poses That Work with Your Theme

Hero Pose! And any poses that take core engagement, focus, and stability. Plank, arm balances, and inversions are also good options.

Distill Your Theme to a Short Sentence or Intention

Be the hero or heroine of your life.

Save yourself.

Phrases or Sentences to Employ in These Parts of Your Class

OPENING	DURING MOVEMENTS
Yoga tells us: Your meandering, anxious mind causes suffering. There is a way to quiet your mind and find peace. The steady and dedicated practice of yoga is that way. Move into our practice today with the intention of quieting your mind and cultivating peace.	Move, knowing that you are making a choice to powerfully embrace the good and peaceful even amidst any darkness or heaviness. You are choosing to define this practice and your life. Feel empowered in this choice. Craft your own narrative of hope and peace.
DURING PAUSES	**CLOSING**
Refusing to be victimized by the circumstances of your life is not necessarily about material changes, but subtle shifts of perspective (that may lead to material changes anyway!). Rest here, and reflect again on your intention to move in ways that empower you and create peace.	You can choose to be a victim of the internal pushing and pulling or you can choose to forge another path. Yoga tells us: The root of your suffering is within you. The path to contentment and peace is within you too. *It's all you.* Whether you suffer or you find peace, the choice is yours. Whatever happens outside your mind, you can cultivate control of your mind and your perspective. What could be more empowering?

Anything Else

For more on the hero's path, read The Bhagavad Gita, and Stephen Cope's lovely book *Yoga and the Quest for the True Self.*

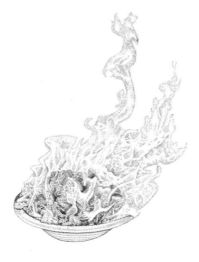

"NEVER STAND UP WHEN YOU CAN SIT DOWN. AND NEVER SIT DOWN WHEN YOU CAN LIE DOWN."

—WINSTON CHURCHILL

Write a Little about Your Theme and Why It Speaks to You

Churchill is said to have attributed his success to "economy of effort," choosing to sit rather than to stand, and to recline when it's possible. For students who are used to applying effort to achieve results, this more languid approach can be a challenge—and a revelation.

Chants, Quotes, Mantras, Poems, or Songs That Connect

Do less.

"Om Shanti" by Daphne Tse

"Not Without Longing" by Karen Benke

Poses That Work with Your Theme

Cue poses that you can do in various relationships to gravity, revealing deeper possibilities for relaxation. Try Eagle Pose and then supine Eagle twists, for instance. Or explore Goddess Squat and then Happy Baby. Show students that they can find the pose but in sweeter, lower energy variations.

Distill Your Theme to a Short Sentence or Intention

Economy of effort.

Do less.

Phrases or Sentences to Employ in These Parts of Your Class

OPENING	DURING MOVEMENTS
Move today with less effort and more ease. Move with an intention to do as little as possible to get into the pose and find the result you seek. Pushing and forcing and so much trying is not the necessary route to success.	Where can you do less? How can you be here with less work? Can you relax your face, your hands?
DURING PAUSES	**CLOSING**
Here is a place of even less effort, a place to unwind further and do even more of doing less.	In Savasana, we practice letting go, knowing it's a practice as important and as serious as fully engaging and working at full energy. As you move out of Corpse Pose, take with you a kernel of this release, and find it again, even as you move into the world with more energy.

Anything Else

Here again we see the power of relaxation. For many students, mustering effort is easy and natural, but letting go is not. Acknowledge that this can be hard!

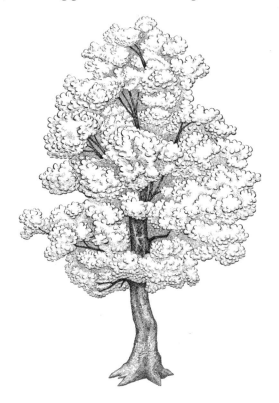

> ·········· "THERE IS A VITALITY, A LIFE FORCE, AN ENERGY, ··········
> A QUICKENING THAT IS TRANSLATED THROUGH
> YOU INTO ACTION, AND BECAUSE THERE IS ONLY
> ONE OF YOU IN ALL OF TIME, THIS EXPRESSION IS
> UNIQUE.... KEEP THE CHANNEL OPEN."
>
> —MARTHA GRAHAM

Write a Little about Your Theme and Why It Speaks to You

The gifted choreographer Martha Graham writes with wisdom here about individual uniqueness. Her quote is a call to arms to not hide individuality and personal spark, but to honor it, revel in it, and above all, allow it to be expressed. For many students, doing yoga and moving their bodies with no apology is the first step toward recognizing and honoring their individuality.

Chants, Quotes, Mantras, Poems, or Songs That Connect

"Thank You" by Alanis Morrisette

"Show Up and Be Heard" by Wah!

"Desiderata" by Max Ehrmann

So hum mantra ("I am")

Poses That Work with Your Theme

Poses that take up space. Five-Pointed Star Pose and Tall Mountain Pose are good options.

Distill Your Theme to a Short Sentence or Intention

There is only one of you.

Keep the channel open.

Phrases or Sentences to Employ in These Parts of Your Class

OPENING	DURING MOVEMENTS
Yoga is the practice of moving your body with intention. Whatever we do in class today, honor your personal approach to the poses. Do this practice remembering that you are a unique being with a unique experience and expression of each pose.	Find a sense of pride in this pose in your body, expressed in a way that no one has ever expressed it before.
DURING PAUSES	**CLOSING**
In a world of homogeneity and conformity, how do you keep your unique channel open? It starts here, in these moments of community with yourself, asking yourself, What do I want? Who am I? How do I walk in this world?	Keep the channel open. There is only one of you. Breathe deeply. Keep the channel open.

Anything Else

We love this reminder that each of us has something special to offer. That's certainly an idea you could explore over a series of classes that highlight different types of poses. This might allow students to identify with the poses that feel uniquely powerful for them.

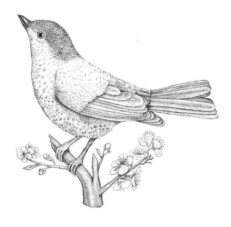

"WHAT IS IT YOU PLAN TO DO WITH YOUR ONE WILD AND PRECIOUS LIFE?"

—MARY OLIVER

Write a Little about Your Theme and Why It Speaks to You

The poem from which this wonderful phrase comes posits that not only is resting in a field in summer not a waste of time, it is time extremely well spent. (This helps people who don't want to do Savasana!) The question is a challenge to live meaningfully, but living meaningfully doesn't always mean *doing* things. It can mean noticing all the beauty and magic of the world. Just noticing and enjoying— wandering a field on a summer day—is a perfect plan for your wild and precious life.

Chants, Quotes, Mantras, Poems, or Songs That Connect

"The Summer Day" by Mary Oliver, from which this line comes.

Do less, have more.

"Slow Dancing in a Burning Room" by John Mayer

Poses That Work with Your Theme

Long holds in luxurious poses, like supine twists.

Distill Your Theme to a Short Sentence or Intention

Enjoy the now.

Phrases or Sentences to Employ in These Parts of Your Class

OPENING	DURING MOVEMENTS
What is it you plan to do with your one wild and precious life? This isn't a call to make lists or plot your future, but a call to enjoy the now and all the beauty around you, while letting all the shoulds and coulds fall away—especially the ones imposed by outside forces. Being fully is doing much.	Are you happy in this pose? This is your wild and precious life in practice. Make this pose a joyful one, by changing whatever you need to change.
DURING PAUSES	**CLOSING**
In rest, so much is happening. Savor the replenishing stillness. Remember that you can stay here for the rest of practice, if you want.	In Savasana, there is nothing to do. There is nothing to do but enjoy the solitude and stillness, the subtle rumblings of your mind in inaction. This is where you should be. Don't wish it away. There is much doing in what appears like doing nothing.

Anything Else

Mary Oliver poems are a continual source of inspiration. She is a poet worth reading in depth.

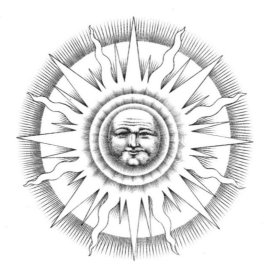

12

BE BASIC, BABY:
OUR FAVORITE SIMPLE IDEAS
THAT RESONATE

UNEXPECTED JOY

Write a Little about Your Theme and Why It Speaks to You

There is extra delight in the unexpected joys. Once you keep your eyes open for them, you'll find them everywhere. Joy can find you in an image, a phrase, a touch. Perhaps you have an eye for four-leafed clovers or heart-shaped rocks. Maybe you delight in a turn of phrase or an unusual but heartfelt complement. Or you could take pleasure in a high-five, fist bump, or shoulder pat. As you appreciate the unexpected joys in daily life, you can also find new wonderful elements of your yoga practice that bring joy: a tiny shift in alignment that feels huge; a particularly sweet exhalation.

Chants, Quotes, Mantras, Poems, or Songs That Connect

"Ode to Joy" by Ludwig Beethoven

"We cannot cure the world of sorrows, but we can choose to live in joy."
—Joseph Campbell

"The Orange" by Wendy Cope

Poses That Work with Your Theme

Any expression of a standing pose with expansive arm movements, like Warrior I with arms spread wide and gaze lifted. Cue playful and releasing breath practices like Breath of Joy, Lion's Breath, or open-mouth sighing.

Distill Your Theme to a Short Sentence or Intention

Look for the unexpected joy.

Phrases or Sentences to Employ in These Parts of Your Class

OPENING	DURING MOVEMENTS
If you've been practicing yoga a long time, it can become rote and overly familiar. As we move today, can you find new things to delight you in unexpected ways? Or, if you're new to practice, everything is unexpected. Can you find joy in the newness?	Where can you find joy here, especially of the unexpected variety? Can you shift your body or your attitude or your approach in and out of the poses to make the experience more joyous?
DURING PAUSES	**CLOSING**
Find the joy in your breath. Find the joy in this moment.	Now that your joy radar is well tuned, listen and look for the unexpected joys throughout your life.

Anything Else

When we find unexpected joy, we share it on social media with the hashtag #ujoy. Join us!

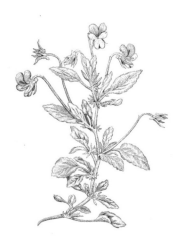

FOCUS (DRISHTI)

Write a Little about Your Theme and Why It Speaks to You

In the practice of *dharana*, or single-pointed focus, *mantra* and *drishti* are both useful. *Drishti*, or the focal point for your gaze, helps you keep your eyes on the prize. Locking your gaze on a nonmoving object confers stability to your poses and helps train your mind to sustain attention over time. *Drishti* is both the physical act of focus and a metaphor for the necessary mental focus it takes to achieve the things we desire.

Chants, Quotes, Mantras, Poems, or Songs That Connect

"Focusing is about saying no." —Steve Jobs

"I Can See for Miles" by The Who

"All I Want" by Joni Mitchell

Poses That Work with Your Theme

All of them! Single-leg standing balance poses are where most students learn the concept and feel the power of *drishti*.

Distill Your Theme to a Short Sentence or Intention

Eyes on the prize.

Phrases or Sentences to Employ in These Parts of Your Class

OPENING	DURING MOVEMENTS
If you've ever ridden a bike, you've learned that your body follows where your gaze is set. As we form intentions for today's practice, set your gaze on a noble goal.	Notice what you're looking at. Could you challenge yourself by changing your *drishti*? Try looking higher, especially in standing poses and single-leg balance poses. And for yet more challenge, close your eyes, if only for a breath. Eyes on the prize.
DURING PAUSES	**CLOSING**
Look inside. Are you moving toward your established goal? Has your focus wavered? Bring it back to your intention.	Look inward and see the divine in you. Open your eyes and see the divine in your classmates. Let's salute that divinity with *namaste*.

Anything Else

As we noted in some of the phrases and sentences you can employ in class, you can teach this theme with a lot of playfulness around *drishti* in balance poses. You could challenge students to close their eyes or choose a *drishti* point on the ceiling, for instance. Another good idea is to explain and demonstrate the pose (Tree, say), and then leave the front of the room so that students practice it without you as their *drishti*.

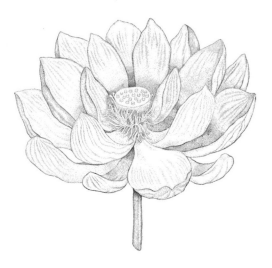

MANTRA

Write a Little about Your Theme and Why It Speaks to You

Mantra means "mind-tool": it is a tool for focusing your mind to sustain attention on one thing over time. A mantra can be quite spiritual, like the mantras we chant in class, or it can be simple or, at first glance, senseless. (If you've ever had the chorus of a song stuck in your head, you know how this can morph into a tool for mental focus.) One of our favorites is *in, out*. This cues and coordinates with the breath, and while the words could seem unimportant, what could be more major than the fact that you are taking this breath, and this one, and this one?

Chants, Quotes, Mantras, Poems, or Songs That Connect

Any mantra at all! Any music that repeats. A good example of this in song form is "Ong Namo" by Martyrs of Sound. The entire song is the repetition of one phrase for over ten minutes. Another is "ReTURNING" by Jennifer Berezan.

Poses That Work with Your Theme

Using mantra as a focus for a meditation practice is a nice way to start or end a class. Balance poses can benefit from the inclusion of mantra as a focusing tool too.

Distill Your Theme to a Short Sentence or Intention

Direct your mind back to the message.

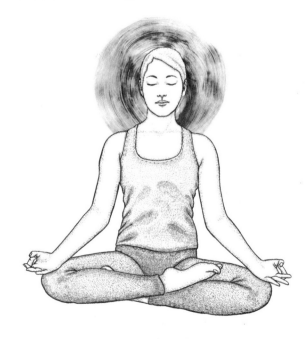

Phrases or Sentences to Employ in These Parts of Your Class

OPENING	DURING MOVEMENTS
Mantra is a focusing tool that can help you on and off your mat. Let's spend the next few moments in silence developing a personal mantra for today's practice. You might start with a word that feels salient today, and add a few words or the opposite word to it, to create a mantra. For instance, if you find peace as your word, you could add "I am" to it: *I am peace.* Or you could explore adding opposite words to magnify your real focus: *Inhale peace, exhale struggle.* Begin to create your mantra now.	As we come into this balance, allow silence in the room to be filled with the mantra you hear in your mind. Let your focus on this mantra create more focus for your balance.
DURING PAUSES	CLOSING
When you're at rest, how does the message of your mantra shift? Do you hear it more clearly here or in movement? Is it more powerful or important to you here or when you're in a space of challenge?	You found a mantra that helped you in your practice today. Take this mantra with you off the mat and into the world. Use it the next time anxiety, fear, or stress arises. See what happens.

Anything Else

It's worth mentioning to students that this isn't just yoga lore; mantra has been researched and has proven to be an effective way to calm and focus the mind. A few resources can be helpful for mantra development. We like Judith Hanson Lasater's book *A Year of Living Your Yoga,* which offers short and thoughtful gems for each day of the year. In addition, using mantra decks like Louise Hay's *Power Thought Cards* can be a fun way for students to explore and create inspiring mantras in a workshop environment.

PRESENCE

Write a Little about Your Theme and Why It Speaks to You

While focus is the ability to sustain attention on one thing over time, presence is the ability to hold your attention on many things simultaneously. Presence, via the mantra "This is what's happening now," is a powerful reminder that the only moment we really have is the one that we're in. When we're present in the moment, we're giving attention to all that is happening *now*—and nothing else.

Chants, Quotes, Mantras, Poems, or Songs That Connect

"The next message you need is always right where you are." —Ram Dass

"Remember then: there is only one time that is important—Now! It is the most important time because it is the only time when we have any power." —Leo Tolstoy

"Be Here Now" by Mason Jennings

Poses That Work with Your Theme

This is a great theme for any class and any poses. It can be especially useful to employ this theme during poses that require a lot of effort.

Distill Your Theme to a Short Sentence or Intention

This is what's happening now. Be here now.

Phrases or Sentences to Employ in These Parts of Your Class

OPENING	DURING MOVEMENTS
The only thing you have to do for the next [number of] minutes is be here and move and breathe. That is your only job. That is the only point. This is what's happening now: you on your mat, making shapes.	Can you be here now? Even if this is a pose you've done a hundred times, can you fully be in the present with the sensations of this pose?
DURING PAUSES	**CLOSING**
In every pause, you get an opportunity to renew your commitment to staying present. Find your breath. Stay present with your breath and with your body at rest on your mat.	Move off your mat with this mantra in your mind: *This is what's happening now.* Come back to this as you find your mind pulling away from the present. It is only in this moment—now—that we have power.

Anything Else

Group yoga classes offer an especially fertile ground for presence, as students get to move away from the mundane distractions of their days and into a sacred space. Practicing presence for sixty, seventy-five, or ninety minutes is a real gift.

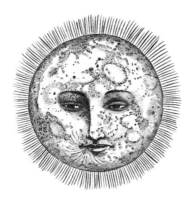

···· BREATH AWARENESS ····

Write a Little about Your Theme and Why It Speaks to You

Your breath reflects your emotions—and it can shape them too. When you become aware of this connection between breath and emotion, you've moved much closer to being able to control your emotional responses—just by changing your breathing! Another key element of breath is that once you've really started paying attention to it—the sensations of breathing, the depth and quality of it—you always have something to pay attention to: you'll never be bored again.

Chants, Quotes, Mantras, Poems, or Songs That Connect

"Breathe In, Breathe Out" by Mat Kearney

"Breathe" by Alexi Murdoch

"Elevator Music" by Henry Taylor

Poses That Work with Your Theme

Restorative poses that allow students to rest in a still space and notice their breathing.

Distill Your Theme to a Short Sentence or Intention

Come back to your breath.

Phrases or Sentences to Employ in These Parts of Your Class

OPENING	DURING MOVEMENTS
Begin to breathe with intention, deepening and slowing your breath. As you settle into stillness, notice where your mind goes. When it leaves this moment and this room, notice and return your attention to your breath.	Even as we move more quickly or begin to focus on a challenging pose, can you keep your breath consistent? Can you be here and stay connected to your breath?
DURING PAUSES	**CLOSING**
Any time we rest in a quiet space, there's an opportunity to come back to the same intentional breath you found at the start of our practice.	Let go of your breath having to do anything. Let your breath come and go. Let your breath come and go.

Anything Else

The Breathing Book by Donna Farhi is an excellent resource for breath work.

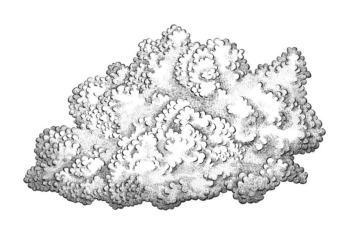

THE OBSTACLE IS THE PATH

Write a Little about Your Theme and Why It Speaks to You

While hindsight is 20/20, often the things we perceive to be major hindrances become our greatest teachers. In the moment, though, when obstacles present themselves, our response is often one of frustration or defeat. Remembering that the obstacle really *is* the path helps us stay true to our heart's calling.

Chants, Quotes, Mantras, Poems, or Songs That Connect

"Only those who dare to fail greatly can ever achieve greatly."
—Robert F. Kennedy

"Keep Breathing" by Ingrid Michaelson

"Driving with Ganesha" by Marti Nikko and DJ Drez

Poses That Work with Your Theme

Arm balances that require several attempts and a positive attitude toward initial failure.

Distill Your Theme to a Short Sentence or Intention

The obstacle is the path. Stay true to your intention, whatever challenge arises.

Phrases or Sentences to Employ in These Parts of Your Class

OPENING	DURING MOVEMENTS
At the start of our day, we often set out to be joyful or to find gratitude. On some days, this comes to fruition. On other days, challenge after challenge presents itself, and maintaining the positive attitude is nearly impossible. The obstacle is always the path. As we move today, look for the ways that challenge tries to throw you off course, whether that's physical challenge or monkey-mind thoughts that disrupt your flow. These obstacles are the teacher. They're the lesson.	Notice what obstacles present as we move into this pose. Does your mind go elsewhere? Is it hard to stay in this pose? What can this challenge offer you?
DURING PAUSES	**CLOSING**
In pauses, the physical challenge of asana is gone, but it's here in this stillness that the mind might recycle old stories or ideas, creating obstacles from within. Notice what your mind tells you here.	As you move off your mat tonight, bring with you the resilience of this practice. Bring with you the memory of overcoming, sustaining, continuing forward despite what arises.

Anything Else

One interesting way to teach this theme is to have students identify some immediate obstacle in their lives during opening meditation. Ask them to revisit it through class, imagining it instead as the only path forward.

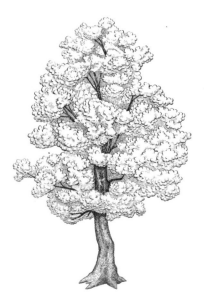

ATTENTION

Write a Little about Your Theme and Why It Speaks to You

Don't think about that white elephant! Of course, now that's all you can notice in your mind. Where we place our attention is where we rest our power. What you put attention on, you grant power. Where you choose to place your attention, then, is a crucial decision. Using "attention" as a theme can serve as an invitation to students to notice where they allow their attention to go throughout class and to recognize that giving attention (or not) is always a choice.

Chants, Quotes, Mantras, Poems, or Songs That Connect

Om Mani Padme Hum mantra

"My experience is what I agree to attend to. Only those items which I notice shape my mind." —William James

"Savasana" by Kamalakar

Poses That Work with Your Theme

Poses that require a lot of attention for success can work nicely here. Consider a balance pose like Hand-to-Big-Toe Pose or a challenging but accessible arm balance, like Flying Pigeon Pose.

Distill Your Theme to a Short Sentence or Intention

Attention is power. Don't give away your attention. Choose where to place it.

Phrases or Sentences to Employ in These Parts of Your Class

OPENING	DURING MOVEMENTS
As we begin, where does your attention immediately go? To your breath? Or does your attention wander to things outside this room, things from earlier in the day or week, things that might happen in the future? Bring your attention back to not only the present, but what you want to focus on now.	To be in this pose, you must offer your attention to the instruction (if it is a new pose for you), and then to each part of your body that is in service in this pose. To be in this pose, you must give attention to your breath. Don't allow your attention to shift to what won't help you here. If you find your attention drawn to what others are doing in this pose, return your attention to where you want it to be.
DURING PAUSES	**CLOSING**
You don't need to spend as much energy on attention in rest: let your mind relax. But watch for ways your relaxation is disrupted by attention that goes to thoughts that create stress or turmoil. Even here, attention matters.	Where you put your attention is a choice, but it's a choice that gets easier to make with practice. Move off your mat and out of the room with attention only to what matters.

Anything Else

Any mindfulness practice grows strong in the continuous guidance of attention back to now. Reassure your students that attention will wander, and that each time they catch it and herd it back to the present moment, they're getting more mindful.

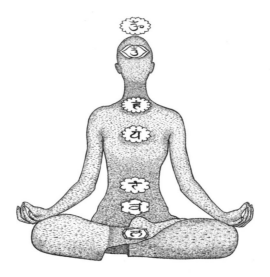

THE POSE BEGINS WHEN YOU WANT TO LEAVE IT

Write a Little about Your Theme and Why It Speaks to You

We have a yoga teacher at our studio who starts his mornings by dumping a bucket of cold water over his head. He does this daily, through the cold of winter to the warmth of summer. His reason for this practice is that the first moment of extreme discomfort, when the cold water touches his skin in the early morning—that moment is the hardest part of his day. Everything else is easier after that. The pose begins when you want to leave it. This may seem like a message primarily regarding physical discomfort, but it's a reminder that enduring *any* discomfort—physical or emotional—gives us a greater ability to endure *future* discomfort. And the truth is that real life has many moments of discomfort that require our presence and attention. We can't always leave discomfort. This theme is the reminder to practice staying with discomfort, on and off the mat. And to bring this point home, you can most definitely start your day with a bucket of cold water (though we do not!).

Chants, Quotes, Mantras, Poems, or Songs That Connect

"When we are able to stay even a moment with uncomfortable energy, we gradually learn not to fear it." —Pema Chödrön

Om Shanti, Shanti, Shanti mantra

"Don't Give Up" by Peter Gabriel with Kate Bush

Poses That Work with Your Theme

Choose poses that are sustainable, but challenging. Lunge poses, but also Pigeon Pose or binds might be good options. Choose slightly longer holds to explore this. A yin yoga practice allows for nice exploration of this theme too.

Distill Your Theme to a Short Sentence or Intention

Stay. See what happens.

Phrases or Sentences to Employ in These Parts of Your Class

OPENING	DURING MOVEMENTS
Let's look at sensation as we move today. When we stay longer in certain poses, and you want to move out of them, what sensations are you experiencing? If there is discomfort due to muscular engagement, can you challenge yourself to stay with the pose for a breath or two longer?	In this pose, practice staying with discomfort. What does your mind tell you about these sensations?
DURING PAUSES	**CLOSING**
The restful spaces in our practice remind us that there is always respite from the challenging moments. There is always relief.	As you settle into the sweet bliss of Savasana, connect again to the challenging moments of our practice that you stayed present for with grace.

Anything Else

The phrase "the pose begins when you want to leave it" or something similar is fairly common in yoga, and it gets attributed to various people. If your students need the reminder, let them know that they should *always* leave a pose if the pose feels unsafe.

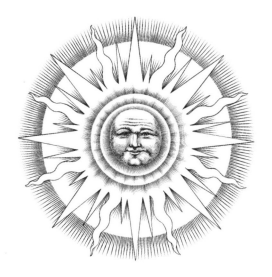

YES, THANKS

Write a Little about Your Theme and Why It Speaks to You

This theme comes to us from Thich Nhat Hanh, and it's a reminder to say *yes* and *thank you* to whatever the present moment has gifted. This theme is about acceptance of what is, now. This theme is about surrendering with acceptance.

Chants, Quotes, Mantras, Poems, or Songs That Connect

"The future is inevitable and precise, but it may not occur. God lurks in the gaps." —Jorge Luis Borges

"Everywhere" by Fleetwood Mac

"Higher Love" performed by James Vincent McMurrow

Poses That Work with Your Theme

Puppy Pose is a beautiful pose of surrender, as is Standing Forward Fold or Wide-Legged Forward Fold (standing or seated).

Distill Your Theme to a Short Sentence or Intention

Yes, thanks.

I accept the now.

Phrases or Sentences to Employ in These Parts of Your Class

OPENING	DURING MOVEMENTS
For this practice, notice any nos or buts that come into your mind, and see if you can inwardly repeat "yes, thanks" instead.	Say "yes, thanks" to the quiver in your legs in Chair Pose. Say "yes, thanks" to the stumble out of Tree Pose.
DURING PAUSES	**CLOSING**
Say "yes, thanks" to this moment of rest. See if you can embrace it the same way you embrace movement.	Now say "yes, thanks" to Savasana. As you move off the mat, practice this mantra of acceptance.

Anything Else

In improvisational theater, a similar concept appears: *yes, and.* We accept what our partner or the world has handed us, and we build on it.

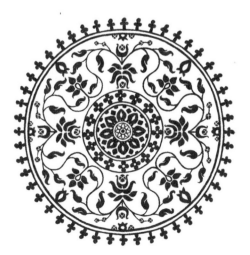

CANCEL AND BLESS

Write a Little about Your Theme and Why It Speaks to You

This theme was gifted to us by a talented yoga teacher, energy healer, performer, and aesthetician who shared that this was one of her favorite mantras. This theme reminds us that we get a chance to forgive—ourselves or others—rather than hold on to anger, recrimination, remorse, or frustration. Cancel and bless is a mantra to employ when someone cuts you off in traffic, and your first thought is *not* charitable. When you notice your mind going toward a dark place, instead cancel the mean thought and send a blessing—cancel and bless. This can work on you yourself too. When you lose your temper or say something foolish—anything that makes you feel remorseful—employ cancel and bless. Forgive yourself; move on.

Chants, Quotes, Mantras, Poems, or Songs That Connect

"Upside Down" by Tori Amos

"Zissou Society Blue Star Cadets/Ned's Theme (Take 1)" by Mark Mothersbaugh

"Muddy water is best cleared by leaving it alone." —Alan Watts

Poses That Work with Your Theme

Balance poses that may be especially challenging. It's useful to employ cancel and bless when you really need it—balance can be a great opportunity to practice letting go and moving on.

Distill Your Theme to a Short Sentence or Intention

Cancel and bless.

Forgive; honor; move on.

Phrases or Sentences to Employ in These Parts of Your Class

OPENING	DURING MOVEMENTS
Every one of us has moments where we think something or say something and instantly regret it. This is human. We can either get stuck in the recrimination or exchange it for a blessing.	Coming back to this pose again, watch your thoughts and look for opportunities to cancel the negative and offer a blessing instead—a blessing for your attempt, a blessing for your ability to be here and challenge yourself.
DURING PAUSES	**CLOSING**
The still spaces give you a chance to feel expansive, free. You are so much more than any negative thought you've ever had.	As we move into Savasana, allow your mind and heart to open to deeper forgiveness—there is nothing to punish yourself over, no regret you have to hold on to here.

Anything Else

We love this twist on *yes, thanks.* It allows for the reactive and negative parts of us, then flips the script toward a more positive, expansive, accepting viewpoint.

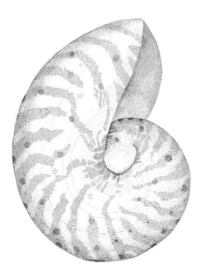

13

INSPIRATION IS EVERYWHERE: THEMES WE LOVE FROM OUTSIDE YOGA

HOW YOU DO ANYTHING IS HOW YOU DO EVERYTHING

Write a Little about Your Theme and Why It Speaks to You

Our yoga mats are laboratories for observing our *samskaras*: the habits we develop and the thought impressions they sear on us. How we move, breathe, think, and feel on the mat is both a reflection of how we do everything in our lives and an opportunity to know better, then do better. Your practice is *darshana:* a lens, a vision of yourself, both as you are and as you can aspire to be. The truism "how you do anything is how you do everything" echoes this yoga wisdom. Your students have likely heard this phrase; it lends itself well to self-study on the mat.

Chants, Quotes, Mantras, Poems, or Songs That Connect

"I Can Change" by Lake Street Dive

"Living" by Denise Levertov

"Wise Up" by Aimee Mann

Poses That Work with Your Theme

All of them! Lead your students through exploration and mindfulness of their habitual patterns on the mat.

Distill Your Theme to a Short Sentence or Intention

As above, so below.

How you do anything is how you do everything.

Phrases or Sentences to Employ in These Parts of Your Class

OPENING	DURING MOVEMENTS
Take your time to get settled here. Imagine someone rushing into the room late, flinging her mat down, and restlessly sighing: is that the energy you want to bring to your practice? Start from a place of centered openness, and your practice will flow from there.	Are you moving fast or slow? Are you pushing too much or not pushing enough? Are you bringing the same energy and movement you've had so far today into your asana practice? And is that the right attitude for now?
DURING PAUSES	**CLOSING**
Notice the thought patterns that arise here. Are you eager to rush to the next movement in the practice? Can you be patient with the rest, with yourself, and by extension, with everyone around you?	Finishing class in this sweet feeling of relaxation, connection, and union gives you a reset to a new launching pad, from where you can move into the world more relaxed, connected, and united. Let how you move in the next few moments dictate how you move in the next after that, and after that. Treat everyone you meet with the same loving kindness you've shown yourself.

Anything Else

The yoga mat is where we can investigate how we do anything and everything, and where we can create helpful new habits that work off the mat. Remind students of this regularly.

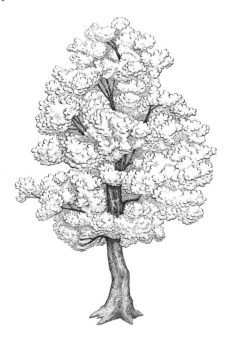

STRESS AND REST

Write a Little about Your Theme and Why It Speaks to You

In sports training, in yoga asana, and most broadly in life, stress is not the enemy: it is the tool for adaptation. Without stress, we would never grow. Stress is the stimulus that encourages us to respond on the cellular and organic levels to become stronger and more resilient. But stress must be met with equal attention to rest, so that the body can recover adequately. (For more on this, see Sage's 2011 book *The Athlete's Guide to Recovery*.) Type-A students are familiar with the stress part of the equation; type B's may be more drawn to the rest side. It's important to find the right balance.

Chants, Quotes, Mantras, Poems, or Songs That Connect

"Krishna Love" by MC Yogi

Om Purnam mantra ("wholeness produces wholeness")

"Funky Guru" by Prem Joshua

Poses That Work with Your Theme

Restorative yoga poses! Try a class with enough movement to let the type A's burn off their upper-end energy, followed by long holds of supported restorative poses.

Distill Your Theme to a Short Sentence or Intention

Moderation in all things.

Phrases or Sentences to Employ in These Parts of Your Class

OPENING	DURING MOVEMENTS
Without stress, we never adapt; with too much stress, we break down. Let's emphasize attention to rest today, as often less is far more for our tissues and our nervous systems.	Make sure you're choosing the right degree of stress here. When in doubt, back off.

DURING PAUSES	CLOSING
Remember that we need to meet our chosen stressors with lots of attention to rest. Notice where you may still be holding on or pushing; instead try to relax as completely as possible. The more you rest here, the more you can push later.	We end class in Savasana, because rest is so critical to our adaptation. Let this Savasana be just the beginning of a different relationship to rest and self-care. How can you slot more rest into your next day, next week, next month?

Anything Else

Sometimes it feels to us, as yoga teachers, that the whole class is a prelude to Savasana. We need to move through the asanas so that we can appreciate the rest at the end to its full value.

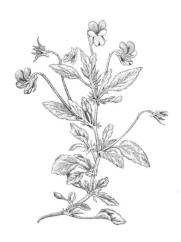

NO CHALLENGE, NO CHANGE

Write a Little about Your Theme and Why It Speaks to You

In the previous theme, we recognized the value of rest. Here, we consider that there has to be challenge for there to be change. If you're looking for transformation, you can't continue with your existing behaviors and expect things to be different. You have to put in the work.

Chants, Quotes, Mantras, Poems, or Songs That Connect

"This is the real meaning of Yoga—a deliverance from contact with pain and sorrow." —B. K. S. Iyengar, introduction, *Light on Yoga*

I can do things that are hard.

"Lift Every Voice" by Lazerbeak

"Love Yourself" by Mary J. Blige

Poses That Work with Your Theme

Navasana (Boat Pose) and other poses that are considered "hard" poses. Core poses in general are a good option. Or take your usual standing sequence and add a level of challenge by having students close their eyes or stand on blocks. (Naturally, you'll want to be sure everyone's safety is paramount.) Or work toward a timed hold of a challenging but safe pose, like Chair Pose or Plank Pose.

Distill Your Theme to a Short Sentence or Intention

No challenge, no change.

If you want to dance, you've got to pay the piper.

Phrases or Sentences to Employ in These Parts of Your Class

OPENING	DURING MOVEMENTS
Consider what it is you would like to change in your practice: your attitude, your ability to breathe under pressure, your amount of time in Crow Pose. Set an intention of embracing the challenge.	Where is the challenge in this movement? Can you keep your effort constant but shift your attitude toward it?
DURING PAUSES	**CLOSING**
Come back to your intention. Recommit to embracing the challenge to create the change.	For the change to take place, you'll need to rest completely so your body can adapt to the challenge you've taken on.

Anything Else

Remember the colloquial definition of insanity: repeating the same behavior and expecting a different outcome. "No challenge, no change" exhorts us to stay sane.

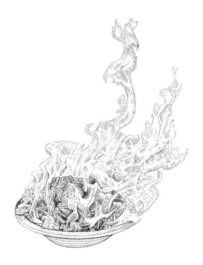

NOT TODAY, MOTHERF——

Write a Little about Your Theme and Why It Speaks to You

This is the opposite of "cancel and bless"! It's a mantra for fierceness and fighting. We were both taken with the story of Kelly Herron, a runner in the Pacific Northwest who, stopping in a public restroom, was attacked and fought off her assailant while deploying this mantra. This is a mantra of protection. It's a mantra to maintain your own power in the face of onslaught.

Chants, Quotes, Mantras, Poems, or Songs That Connect

"I Won't Back Down" by Tom Petty and the Heartbreakers

"This world is the gymnasium where we come to make ourselves strong." —Swami Vivekananda

Om Gam Ganapataye Namah mantra (Salutations to Ganesh, remover of obstacles)

Poses That Work with Your Theme

Poses that require focus and fierceness. Consider Warrior III and variations on High Lunge.

Distill Your Theme to a Short Sentence or Intention

Not today.

I am strong.

Phrases or Sentences to Employ in These Parts of Your Class

OPENING	DURING MOVEMENTS
Often we walk about the world allowing others to define our emotions. We get ping-ponged by a bad driver or a rude checkout clerk or a tense interaction at work. "Not today, motherf——" is a reminder that your locus of control is internal, despite external forces. Move today with an intention to stay present with yourself. Look for ways you get pulled away. And when you see those ways, remind yourself: not today.	Don't just do this pose; bring your full fierceness to it. Bring your power and your strength.
DURING PAUSES	CLOSING
Regroup, go deep, and listen to your heart your mind, your body. Your strength is here.	Move off your mat with a renewed appreciation for your own internal power. You are strong.

Anything Else

While many of our themes and much of yoga philosophy is about accepting what is, this mantra is a fierce reminder that sometimes action is necessary. The Bhagavad Gita makes the same point, and you might make that connection for your students. Krishna's message to Arjuna is about the necessity of action.

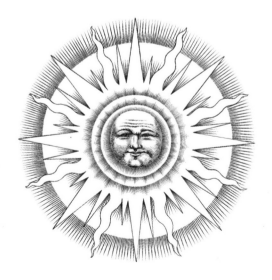

OWN YOUR POWER

Write a Little about Your Theme and Why It Speaks to You

"Own your own power" is a reminder that we often undersell ourselves or imagine that we're still some past (demurer or more cautious) version of ourselves. "Own your own power" isn't a call to ego; it's a call to self-empowerment that can create real change in the world. "Own your own power" is about recognizing all the power you already possess, right now, today.

Chants, Quotes, Mantras, Poems, or Songs That Connect

"Song of Myself" by Walt Whitman

"Respect Yourself" by the Staple Singers

"Be the Change" by MC Yogi

Poses That Work with Your Theme

Goddess Pose, Warrior poses, Chair Pose, Plank, Side Plank

Distill Your Theme to a Short Sentence or Intention

Own your power.

Phrases or Sentences to Employ in These Parts of Your Class

OPENING	DURING MOVEMENTS
As you move into practice today, do so believing that you can do all parts of the practice offered. Move into class today without undermining yourself in advance of the poses we'll explore. Move with the knowledge of your own strength, your own power.	Owning your power doesn't mean moving unsafely; take rest or modifications that allow you to move with ease and grace. But if you modify and rest, do it with a sense of ownership, not apology. If you rest, rest because you know your limits and you're wisely obeying them, not because you've been defeated by anything.
DURING PAUSES	CLOSING
In rest, you cultivate the strength to shine again.	Own your power. Go into the world with this memory of the freedom of empowerment and deserved self-confidence. Make no apologies.

Anything Else

Teaching this along with *asmita* can be an enlightening theme. Students can begin to differentiate between ego and self-worth derived from within.

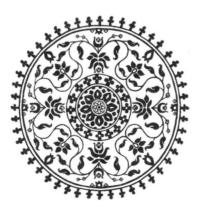

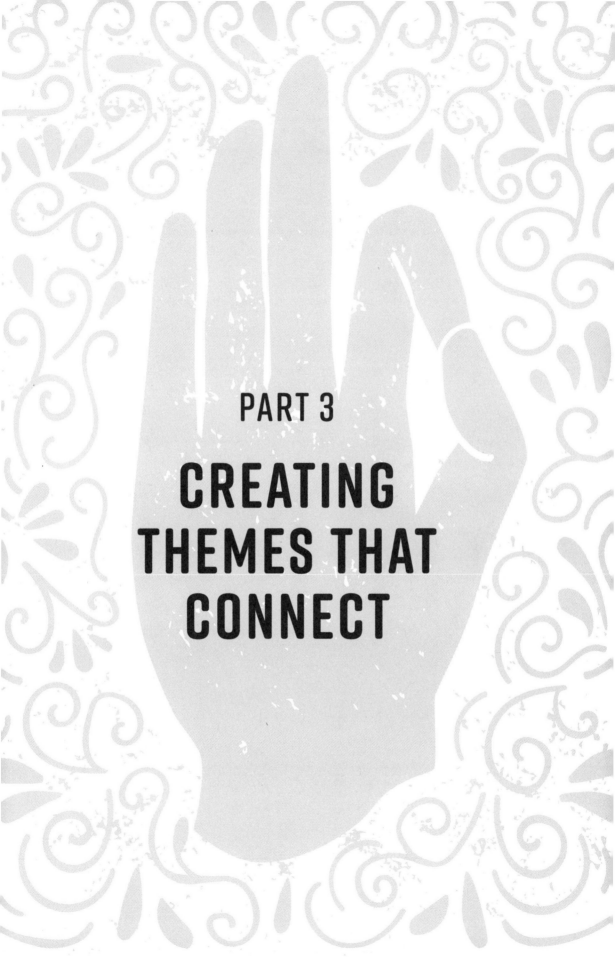

PART 3

CREATING THEMES THAT CONNECT

14

THERE ARE NO BAD THEMES: JUST WRITE IT DOWN

As you create your own themes, emphasize progress over perfection. Sometimes getting started is the hardest part! All writers are familiar with writer's block. We know it well too. The trick is to get started. Don't feel like you need to create much of value; just begin. Put pen to the page and start.

An exercise from writing class might help: freewriting. In freewriting, you set a timer and start writing (or typing) continuously for the duration of your timer. Write whatever comes into your head—it doesn't have to be good, or even be complete sentences, but just keep writing. You might come up with something like:

> Theme. Theme. Scream. I can't think of what to say nothing is coming to mind perhaps there could be a theme about how tough theming is. About the importance of being present for creativity to happen—that we have to get on the mat even in times when we don't feel like it, and sometimes inspiration strikes. The same is true for writing. Sometimes having a set sequence to move through like Sun Salutations or a familiar warmup is good. The ritual gets us rolling. But ritual can get stale and lifeless with time....

Sometimes the act of getting started generates its own momentum, and you're able to continue to work on a theme that will make it into your class planning. Other times, you'll create a page or more of freewriting and then need to walk away from it. In a day, or a week, take another look and see whether what you've written has any seeds in it that you can grow into something bigger.

⸻ DEADLINES AND ACCOUNTABILITY ⸻

There's nothing like a deadline to get you motivated! While you may have every good intention to create a journal full of well-considered themes, that doesn't happen in a vacuum. You need to have a time-specific goal to work toward, and it's helpful to have someone to hold you accountable. You're answering to your class of students, of course, but having a peer group, a teaching partner, or a mentor to bounce your ideas off can help you refine and grow in new ways.

Try forming an accountability group, either virtually or in person. Set a monthly or bimonthly meet-up and share your work. This can happen at your home studio, which offers a good chance to strengthen both individual teachers' classes and the studio brand as a whole. Or get collegially collaborative: invite all local teachers to join the group, and rotate home base among all the local studios. Or form a yoga teacher's group through social media, where you can all share your theming inspiration and borrow each other's good ideas! We have also established a community for sharing themes at http://teachingyogabeyondtheposes.com.

Or if working alone is more your speed, be sure that you set aside specific time in your week to plan your yoga class themes (and sequences), so that you always have this time accounted for and you dedicate your energy to the task of good theming. If you even dedicate one hour to this weekly, you'll create four strong themes each month. That's a theme a week to help you stay fresh and bring new inspiration to your students regularly.

15

INSPIRATIONAL PROMPTS FOR CREATING THEMES

In this section, we have space for readers to create lists of songs, chants, poems, quotes, and mantras that they can revisit and flush out into theme form—and we also provide a list of themes that can easily be expanded, such as theming around body parts or theming connected to holidays (traditional and nontraditional.) We also have journal-type prompts that help teachers and home practitioners instantly get inspired and carry that inspiration to others.

The very best themes are the ones you'll come up with on your own. When you're speaking completely with your voice on the topics that best resonate with you, your authenticity shines through. Find some inspiration in the prompts here, and every time you notice a germ of a new theme, be sure to write it down for future expansion.

CONCEPTS TO EXPAND

These concepts appear frequently in yoga class—you may even hear yourself mentioning them naturally in the course of your cueing. Each could be expanded to a full theme. Add to our list with other ideas of your own.

- open heart
- letting go
- getting grounded
- roots and wings
- fear of flying
- hug inward
- radiate outward
- listen to your body

BODY PARTS AND ACTIONS

Paying attention to a particular region of the body, or to a kinesthetic action the body can make, can lead to a new theme. These work particularly well as a focus of the month, or as inspiration for a limited series of three to six classes. Add your own.

- the feet
- the knees
- the hips
- the lower back
- the upper back
- the shoulders
- the arms
- the core
- the neck
- forward folding
- back bending
- twisting
- side bending
- inversions

HOLIDAYS

We both teach a regular Monday class, which means we often find ourselves including the reason for the holiday as part of our theme. Add your own holidays and notes.

- New Year's Day: setting intentions, awakening to newness
- Martin Luther King Jr. Day: connection, community, justice
- Valentine's Day: a celebration of love as the root of everything
- Presidents' Day: leadership, ethics
- Easter: new growth, new life, self-sacrifice
- Holi: spring, revelry, and joyful merrymaking
- Earth Day: grounding theme, mention of Gaia
- Arbor Day: Tree Pose, growing your branches
- Mother's Day: appreciation of the creator, divine feminine
- Memorial Day: Warrior poses, mention of Arjuna's fight in The Bhagavad Gita
- Eid Al-Fitr: generosity, empathy, charity
- Father's Day: appreciation of role models, divine masculine
- Independence Day: freedom, interdependence
- Labor Day: recognition of the work we do, and the importance of also taking rest
- Yom Kippur: forgiveness, release
- Columbus Day/Indigenous Peoples' Day: exploration, appreciation of traditions
- Veterans Day: appreciation of peace, surrender
- Halloween: poses that scare you, Cat Pose, Corpse Pose
- Diwali: celebrating good's triumph over evil, lightness
- Thanksgiving: gratitude, bounty, family
- Hanukkah: light in the darkness, our ability to sustain beyond our perceived limits
- Christmas: the gift of hope
- New Year's Eve: reflection on the past year, release of the old to make room for the new

JOURNALING PROMPTS

Let these prompts lead you to some freeform writing, from which a theme can emerge.

A common thread in my best classes is …

My students tell me they appreciate …

I love it when my teachers …

The most memorable yoga class I ever attended taught me …

The most frustrating yoga class I ever attended taught me …

Three words that sum up my intention as a teacher are …

A major theme in my yoga journey has been …

One theme that I still need to hear is …

If I had to explain why I love yoga, I'd say …

One idea from yoga I still want to learn more about is …

16

TEMPLATES FOR THEMING ANY STYLE OF CLASS

Now create your own themes. As you do, feel free to add additional sections, omit aspects that don't apply to your teaching style, and change anything you want! You can also download a template in your favorite file format at http:// teachingyogabeyondtheposes.com.

THEME NAME

Write a Little about Your Theme and Why It Speaks to You

Chants, Quotes, Mantras, Poems, or Songs That Connect

Poses That Work with Your Theme

Distill Your Theme to a Short Sentence or Intention

Phrases or Sentences to Employ in These Parts of Your Class

OPENING	DURING MOVEMENTS
DURING PAUSES	**CLOSING**

Anything Else

THEME NAME

Write a Little about Your Theme and Why It Speaks to You

Chants, Quotes, Mantras, Poems, or Songs That Connect

Poses That Work with Your Theme

Distill Your Theme to a Short Sentence or Intention

Phrases or Sentences to Employ in These Parts of Your Class

OPENING	DURING MOVEMENTS
DURING PAUSES	**CLOSING**

Anything Else

THEME NAME

Write a Little about Your Theme and Why It Speaks to You

Chants, Quotes, Mantras, Poems, or Songs That Connect

Poses That Work with Your Theme

Distill Your Theme to a Short Sentence or Intention

Phrases or Sentences to Employ in These Parts of Your Class

OPENING	DURING MOVEMENTS
DURING PAUSES	CLOSING

Anything Else

THEME NAME

Write a Little about Your Theme and Why It Speaks to You

Chants, Quotes, Mantras, Poems, or Songs That Connect

Poses That Work with Your Theme

Distill Your Theme to a Short Sentence or Intention

Phrases or Sentences to Employ in These Parts of Your Class

OPENING	DURING MOVEMENTS
DURING PAUSES	CLOSING

Anything Else

THEME NAME

Write a Little about Your Theme and Why It Speaks to You

Chants, Quotes, Mantras, Poems, or Songs That Connect

Poses That Work with Your Theme

Distill Your Theme to a Short Sentence or Intention

Phrases or Sentences to Employ in These Parts of Your Class

OPENING	DURING MOVEMENTS
DURING PAUSES	CLOSING

Anything Else

THEME NAME

Write a Little about Your Theme and Why It Speaks to You

Chants, Quotes, Mantras, Poems, or Songs That Connect

Poses That Work with Your Theme

Distill Your Theme to a Short Sentence or Intention

Phrases or Sentences to Employ in These Parts of Your Class

OPENING	DURING MOVEMENTS
DURING PAUSES	CLOSING

Anything Else

THEME NAME

Write a Little about Your Theme and Why It Speaks to You

Chants, Quotes, Mantras, Poems, or Songs That Connect

Poses That Work with Your Theme

Distill Your Theme to a Short Sentence or Intention

Phrases or Sentences to Employ in These Parts of Your Class

OPENING	DURING MOVEMENTS
DURING PAUSES	**CLOSING**

Anything Else

THEME NAME

Write a Little about Your Theme and Why It Speaks to You

Chants, Quotes, Mantras, Poems, or Songs That Connect

Poses That Work with Your Theme

Distill Your Theme to a Short Sentence or Intention

Phrases or Sentences to Employ in These Parts of Your Class

OPENING	DURING MOVEMENTS
DURING PAUSES	CLOSING

Anything Else

THEME NAME

Write a Little about Your Theme and Why It Speaks to You

Chants, Quotes, Mantras, Poems, or Songs That Connect

Poses That Work with Your Theme

Distill Your Theme to a Short Sentence or Intention

Phrases or Sentences to Employ in These Parts of Your Class

OPENING	DURING MOVEMENTS
DURING PAUSES	CLOSING

Anything Else

THEME NAME

Write a Little about Your Theme and Why It Speaks to You

Chants, Quotes, Mantras, Poems, or Songs That Connect

Poses That Work with Your Theme

Distill Your Theme to a Short Sentence or Intention

Phrases or Sentences to Employ in These Parts of Your Class

OPENING	DURING MOVEMENTS
DURING PAUSES	**CLOSING**

Anything Else

THEME NAME

Write a Little about Your Theme and Why It Speaks to You

Chants, Quotes, Mantras, Poems, or Songs That Connect

Poses That Work with Your Theme

Distill Your Theme to a Short Sentence or Intention

Phrases or Sentences to Employ in These Parts of Your Class

OPENING	DURING MOVEMENTS
DURING PAUSES	**CLOSING**

Anything Else

THEME NAME

Write a Little about Your Theme and Why It Speaks to You

Chants, Quotes, Mantras, Poems, or Songs That Connect

Poses That Work with Your Theme

Distill Your Theme to a Short Sentence or Intention

Phrases or Sentences to Employ in These Parts of Your Class

OPENING	DURING MOVEMENTS
DURING PAUSES	CLOSING

Anything Else

THEME NAME

Write a Little about Your Theme and Why It Speaks to You

Chants, Quotes, Mantras, Poems, or Songs That Connect

Poses That Work with Your Theme

Distill Your Theme to a Short Sentence or Intention

Phrases or Sentences to Employ in These Parts of Your Class

OPENING	DURING MOVEMENTS
DURING PAUSES	**CLOSING**

Anything Else

THEME NAME

Write a Little about Your Theme and Why It Speaks to You

Chants, Quotes, Mantras, Poems, or Songs That Connect

Poses That Work with Your Theme

Distill Your Theme to a Short Sentence or Intention

Phrases or Sentences to Employ in These Parts of Your Class

OPENING	DURING MOVEMENTS
DURING PAUSES	CLOSING

Anything Else

THEME NAME

Write a Little about Your Theme and Why It Speaks to You

Chants, Quotes, Mantras, Poems, or Songs That Connect

Poses That Work with Your Theme

Distill Your Theme to a Short Sentence or Intention

Phrases or Sentences to Employ in These Parts of Your Class

OPENING	DURING MOVEMENTS
DURING PAUSES	CLOSING

Anything Else

THEME NAME

Write a Little about Your Theme and Why It Speaks to You

Chants, Quotes, Mantras, Poems, or Songs That Connect

Poses That Work with Your Theme

Distill Your Theme to a Short Sentence or Intention

Phrases or Sentences to Employ in These Parts of Your Class

OPENING	DURING MOVEMENTS
DURING PAUSES	CLOSING

Anything Else

THEME NAME

Write a Little about Your Theme and Why It Speaks to You

Chants, Quotes, Mantras, Poems, or Songs That Connect

Poses That Work with Your Theme

Distill Your Theme to a Short Sentence or Intention

Phrases or Sentences to Employ in These Parts of Your Class

OPENING	DURING MOVEMENTS
DURING PAUSES	CLOSING

Anything Else

THEME NAME

Write a Little about Your Theme and Why It Speaks to You

Chants, Quotes, Mantras, Poems, or Songs That Connect

Poses That Work with Your Theme

Distill Your Theme to a Short Sentence or Intention

Phrases or Sentences to Employ in These Parts of Your Class

OPENING	DURING MOVEMENTS
DURING PAUSES	CLOSING

Anything Else

THEME NAME

Write a Little about Your Theme and Why It Speaks to You

Chants, Quotes, Mantras, Poems, or Songs That Connect

Poses That Work with Your Theme

Distill Your Theme to a Short Sentence or Intention

Phrases or Sentences to Employ in These Parts of Your Class

OPENING	DURING MOVEMENTS
DURING PAUSES	CLOSING

Anything Else

THEME NAME

Write a Little about Your Theme and Why It Speaks to You

Chants, Quotes, Mantras, Poems, or Songs That Connect

Poses That Work with Your Theme

Distill Your Theme to a Short Sentence or Intention

Phrases or Sentences to Employ in These Parts of Your Class

OPENING	DURING MOVEMENTS
DURING PAUSES	CLOSING

Anything Else

···· THEME NAME ····

Write a Little about Your Theme and Why It Speaks to You

.

Chants, Quotes, Mantras, Poems, or Songs That Connect

Poses That Work with Your Theme

Distill Your Theme to a Short Sentence or Intention

Phrases or Sentences to Employ in These Parts of Your Class

OPENING	DURING MOVEMENTS
DURING PAUSES	CLOSING

Anything Else

THEME NAME

Write a Little about Your Theme and Why It Speaks to You

Chants, Quotes, Mantras, Poems, or Songs That Connect

Poses That Work with Your Theme

Distill Your Theme to a Short Sentence or Intention

Phrases or Sentences to Employ in These Parts of Your Class

OPENING	DURING MOVEMENTS
DURING PAUSES	CLOSING

Anything Else

THEME NAME

Write a Little about Your Theme and Why It Speaks to You

Chants, Quotes, Mantras, Poems, or Songs That Connect

Poses That Work with Your Theme

Distill Your Theme to a Short Sentence or Intention

Phrases or Sentences to Employ in These Parts of Your Class

OPENING	DURING MOVEMENTS
DURING PAUSES	CLOSING

Anything Else

THEME NAME

Write a Little about Your Theme and Why It Speaks to You

Chants, Quotes, Mantras, Poems, or Songs That Connect

Poses That Work with Your Theme

Distill Your Theme to a Short Sentence or Intention

Phrases or Sentences to Employ in These Parts of Your Class

OPENING	DURING MOVEMENTS
DURING PAUSES	CLOSING

Anything Else

THEME NAME

Write a Little about Your Theme and Why It Speaks to You

Chants, Quotes, Mantras, Poems, or Songs That Connect

Poses That Work with Your Theme

Distill Your Theme to a Short Sentence or Intention

Phrases or Sentences to Employ in These Parts of Your Class

OPENING	DURING MOVEMENTS
DURING PAUSES	CLOSING

Anything Else

THEME NAME

Write a Little about Your Theme and Why It Speaks to You

Chants, Quotes, Mantras, Poems, or Songs That Connect

Poses That Work with Your Theme

Distill Your Theme to a Short Sentence or Intention

Phrases or Sentences to Employ in These Parts of Your Class

OPENING	DURING MOVEMENTS
DURING PAUSES	CLOSING

Anything Else

THEME NAME

Write a Little about Your Theme and Why It Speaks to You

Chants, Quotes, Mantras, Poems, or Songs That Connect

Poses That Work with Your Theme

Distill Your Theme to a Short Sentence or Intention

Phrases or Sentences to Employ in These Parts of Your Class

OPENING	DURING MOVEMENTS
DURING PAUSES	**CLOSING**

Anything Else

THEME NAME

Write a Little about Your Theme and Why It Speaks to You

Chants, Quotes, Mantras, Poems, or Songs That Connect

Poses That Work with Your Theme

Distill Your Theme to a Short Sentence or Intention

Phrases or Sentences to Employ in These Parts of Your Class

OPENING	DURING MOVEMENTS
DURING PAUSES	CLOSING

Anything Else

···················· THEME NAME ····················

Write a Little about Your Theme and Why It Speaks to You

Chants, Quotes, Mantras, Poems, or Songs That Connect

Poses That Work with Your Theme

Distill Your Theme to a Short Sentence or Intention

Phrases or Sentences to Employ in These Parts of Your Class

OPENING	DURING MOVEMENTS
DURING PAUSES	**CLOSING**

Anything Else

THEME NAME

Write a Little about Your Theme and Why It Speaks to You

Chants, Quotes, Mantras, Poems, or Songs That Connect

Poses That Work with Your Theme

Distill Your Theme to a Short Sentence or Intention

Phrases or Sentences to Employ in These Parts of Your Class

OPENING	DURING MOVEMENTS
DURING PAUSES	CLOSING

Anything Else

THEME NAME

Write a Little about Your Theme and Why It Speaks to You

Chants, Quotes, Mantras, Poems, or Songs That Connect

Poses That Work with Your Theme

Distill Your Theme to a Short Sentence or Intention

Phrases or Sentences to Employ in These Parts of Your Class

OPENING	DURING MOVEMENTS
DURING PAUSES	CLOSING

Anything Else

THEME NAME

Write a Little about Your Theme and Why It Speaks to You

Chants, Quotes, Mantras, Poems, or Songs That Connect

Poses That Work with Your Theme

Distill Your Theme to a Short Sentence or Intention

Phrases or Sentences to Employ in These Parts of Your Class

OPENING	DURING MOVEMENTS
DURING PAUSES	CLOSING

Anything Else

THEME NAME

Write a Little about Your Theme and Why It Speaks to You

Chants, Quotes, Mantras, Poems, or Songs That Connect

Poses That Work with Your Theme

Distill Your Theme to a Short Sentence or Intention

Phrases or Sentences to Employ in These Parts of Your Class

OPENING	DURING MOVEMENTS
DURING PAUSES	CLOSING

Anything Else

THEME NAME

Write a Little about Your Theme and Why It Speaks to You

Chants, Quotes, Mantras, Poems, or Songs That Connect

Poses That Work with Your Theme

Distill Your Theme to a Short Sentence or Intention

Phrases or Sentences to Employ in These Parts of Your Class

OPENING	DURING MOVEMENTS
DURING PAUSES	**CLOSING**

Anything Else

THEME NAME

Write a Little about Your Theme and Why It Speaks to You

Chants, Quotes, Mantras, Poems, or Songs That Connect

Poses That Work with Your Theme

Distill Your Theme to a Short Sentence or Intention

Phrases or Sentences to Employ in These Parts of Your Class

OPENING	DURING MOVEMENTS
DURING PAUSES	CLOSING

Anything Else

THEME NAME

Write a Little about Your Theme and Why It Speaks to You

Chants, Quotes, Mantras, Poems, or Songs That Connect

Poses That Work with Your Theme

Distill Your Theme to a Short Sentence or Intention

Phrases or Sentences to Employ in These Parts of Your Class

OPENING	DURING MOVEMENTS
DURING PAUSES	CLOSING

Anything Else

THEME NAME

Write a Little about Your Theme and Why It Speaks to You

Chants, Quotes, Mantras, Poems, or Songs That Connect

Poses That Work with Your Theme

Distill Your Theme to a Short Sentence or Intention

Phrases or Sentences to Employ in These Parts of Your Class

OPENING	DURING MOVEMENTS
DURING PAUSES	CLOSING

Anything Else

THEME NAME

Write a Little about Your Theme and Why It Speaks to You

Chants, Quotes, Mantras, Poems, or Songs That Connect

Poses That Work with Your Theme

Distill Your Theme to a Short Sentence or Intention

Phrases or Sentences to Employ in These Parts of Your Class

OPENING	DURING MOVEMENTS
DURING PAUSES	CLOSING

Anything Else

THEME NAME

Write a Little about Your Theme and Why It Speaks to You

Chants, Quotes, Mantras, Poems, or Songs That Connect

Poses That Work with Your Theme

Distill Your Theme to a Short Sentence or Intention

Phrases or Sentences to Employ in These Parts of Your Class

OPENING	DURING MOVEMENTS
DURING PAUSES	CLOSING

Anything Else

THEME NAME

Write a Little about Your Theme and Why It Speaks to You

Chants, Quotes, Mantras, Poems, or Songs That Connect

Poses That Work with Your Theme

Distill Your Theme to a Short Sentence or Intention

Phrases or Sentences to Employ in These Parts of Your Class

OPENING	DURING MOVEMENTS
DURING PAUSES	CLOSING

Anything Else

THEME NAME

Write a Little about Your Theme and Why It Speaks to You

Chants, Quotes, Mantras, Poems, or Songs That Connect

Poses That Work with Your Theme

Distill Your Theme to a Short Sentence or Intention

Phrases or Sentences to Employ in These Parts of Your Class

OPENING	DURING MOVEMENTS
DURING PAUSES	CLOSING

Anything Else

THEME NAME

Write a Little about Your Theme and Why It Speaks to You

Chants, Quotes, Mantras, Poems, or Songs That Connect

Poses That Work with Your Theme

Distill Your Theme to a Short Sentence or Intention

Phrases or Sentences to Employ in These Parts of Your Class

OPENING	DURING MOVEMENTS
DURING PAUSES	**CLOSING**

Anything Else

THEME NAME

Write a Little about Your Theme and Why It Speaks to You

Chants, Quotes, Mantras, Poems, or Songs That Connect

Poses That Work with Your Theme

Distill Your Theme to a Short Sentence or Intention

Phrases or Sentences to Employ in These Parts of Your Class

OPENING	DURING MOVEMENTS
DURING PAUSES	CLOSING

Anything Else

THEME NAME

Write a Little about Your Theme and Why It Speaks to You

Chants, Quotes, Mantras, Poems, or Songs That Connect

Poses That Work with Your Theme

Distill Your Theme to a Short Sentence or Intention

Phrases or Sentences to Employ in These Parts of Your Class

OPENING	DURING MOVEMENTS
DURING PAUSES	**CLOSING**

Anything Else

THEME NAME

Write a Little about Your Theme and Why It Speaks to You

Chants, Quotes, Mantras, Poems, or Songs That Connect

Poses That Work with Your Theme

Distill Your Theme to a Short Sentence or Intention

Phrases or Sentences to Employ in These Parts of Your Class

OPENING	DURING MOVEMENTS
DURING PAUSES	CLOSING

Anything Else

THEME NAME

Write a Little about Your Theme and Why It Speaks to You

Chants, Quotes, Mantras, Poems, or Songs That Connect

Poses That Work with Your Theme

Distill Your Theme to a Short Sentence or Intention

Phrases or Sentences to Employ in These Parts of Your Class

OPENING	DURING MOVEMENTS
DURING PAUSES	**CLOSING**

Anything Else

THEME NAME

Write a Little about Your Theme and Why It Speaks to You

Chants, Quotes, Mantras, Poems, or Songs That Connect

Poses That Work with Your Theme

Distill Your Theme to a Short Sentence or Intention

Phrases or Sentences to Employ in These Parts of Your Class

OPENING	DURING MOVEMENTS
DURING PAUSES	CLOSING

Anything Else

THEME NAME

Write a Little about Your Theme and Why It Speaks to You

Chants, Quotes, Mantras, Poems, or Songs That Connect

Poses That Work with Your Theme

Distill Your Theme to a Short Sentence or Intention

Phrases or Sentences to Employ in These Parts of Your Class

OPENING	DURING MOVEMENTS
DURING PAUSES	CLOSING

Anything Else

THEME NAME

Write a Little about Your Theme and Why It Speaks to You

Chants, Quotes, Mantras, Poems, or Songs That Connect

Poses That Work with Your Theme

Distill Your Theme to a Short Sentence or Intention

Phrases or Sentences to Employ in These Parts of Your Class

OPENING	DURING MOVEMENTS
DURING PAUSES	**CLOSING**

Anything Else

THEME NAME

Write a Little about Your Theme and Why It Speaks to You

Chants, Quotes, Mantras, Poems, or Songs That Connect

Poses That Work with Your Theme

Distill Your Theme to a Short Sentence or Intention

Phrases or Sentences to Employ in These Parts of Your Class

OPENING	DURING MOVEMENTS
DURING PAUSES	**CLOSING**

Anything Else

THEME NAME

Write a Little about Your Theme and Why It Speaks to You

Chants, Quotes, Mantras, Poems, or Songs That Connect

Poses That Work with Your Theme

Distill Your Theme to a Short Sentence or Intention

Phrases or Sentences to Employ in These Parts of Your Class

OPENING	DURING MOVEMENTS
DURING PAUSES	**CLOSING**

Anything Else

THEME NAME

Write a Little about Your Theme and Why It Speaks to You

Chants, Quotes, Mantras, Poems, or Songs That Connect

Poses That Work with Your Theme

Distill Your Theme to a Short Sentence or Intention

Phrases or Sentences to Employ in These Parts of Your Class

OPENING	DURING MOVEMENTS
DURING PAUSES	CLOSING

Anything Else

⋯⋯⋯ THEME NAME ⋯⋯⋯

Write a Little about Your Theme and Why It Speaks to You

Chants, Quotes, Mantras, Poems, or Songs That Connect

Poses That Work with Your Theme

Distill Your Theme to a Short Sentence or Intention

Phrases or Sentences to Employ in These Parts of Your Class

OPENING	DURING MOVEMENTS
DURING PAUSES	**CLOSING**

Anything Else

THEME NAME

Write a Little about Your Theme and Why It Speaks to You

Chants, Quotes, Mantras, Poems, or Songs That Connect

Poses That Work with Your Theme

Distill Your Theme to a Short Sentence or Intention

Phrases or Sentences to Employ in These Parts of Your Class

OPENING	DURING MOVEMENTS
DURING PAUSES	CLOSING

Anything Else